Urban Health Issues

Urban Health Issues

Exploring the Impacts of Big-City Living

Richard V. Crume

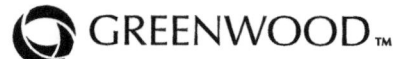

GREENWOOD™

An Imprint of ABC-CLIO, LLC
Santa Barbara, California • Denver, Colorado

Library of Congress Cataloging-in-Publication Data

Names: Crume, Richard V., author.
Title: Urban health issues : exploring the impacts of big-city living / Richard Crume.
Description: Santa Barbara, CA : Greenwood, [2019] | Includes bibliographical references and index.
Identifiers: LCCN 2018053928 (print) | LCCN 2019000048 (ebook) |
  ISBN 9781440861727 (ebook) | ISBN 9781440861710 (hard copy : alk. paper)
Subjects: LCSH: Urban health.
Classification: LCC RA566.7 (ebook) | LCC RA566.7 .C78 2019 (print) |
  DDC 362.1/042—dc23
LC record available at https://lccn.loc.gov/2018053928

ISBN: 978-1-4408-6171-0 (print)
    978-1-4408-6172-7 (ebook)

23 22 21 20 19   1 2 3 4 5

This book is also available as an eBook.

Greenwood
An Imprint of ABC-CLIO, LLC

ABC-CLIO, LLC
147 Castilian Drive
Santa Barbara, California 93117
www.abc-clio.com

This book is printed on acid-free paper ∞

Manufactured in the United States of America

This work is dedicated to the 25,000 members of the American Public Health Association, championing the health of all people, speaking out for public health issues and policies backed by science, and working to eliminate disparities in healthcare quality and access. With a history spanning 150 years, the association represents the concerns of professionals from all disciplines of public health in over 40 countries.

Contents

Preface

Urban health is a broad and complex topic encompassing a wide variety of concerns, ranging from environmental pollution and the spread of infectious diseases to drug and alcohol abuse and the importance of social support networks. Even climate change, a global phenomenon, has a direct effect on the health of urban dwellers. To cover these complexities in a single volume, a three-pronged strategy has been employed involving entries on topics central to the study of urban health, commentaries by global health experts on the latest urban health concerns, and case studies highlighting the innovative approaches that many cities are taking to provide a healthy living and working environment. Each entry includes sections on health issues and concerns, relevant city initiatives, and recommendations for urban dwellers. Additionally, a historical perspective on urban health is provided, along with a discussion of steps that city residents can follow for healthy urban living. A glossary and directory of resources are included as well.

Rather than reading this entire work in one sitting, most readers will probably be interested in investigating just one topic or several topics at a time. Because the expert commentaries and case studies are interspersed among the specific entries they are related to (e.g., the case study on healthcare delivery in Delhi is included with the "Healthcare Access and Quality" entry), there is no need to search multiple sections of the book to find all of the information related to a given topic. Instead, the reader need only review the entry on a particular topic of interest.

As the world becomes more urbanized, providing a healthy urban environment has become a leading issue of the twenty-first century, and how cities respond to this challenge will determine the fate of potentially hundreds of millions of global inhabitants. In preparing this work, my goal was to help urban dwellers and health professionals understand the complexities of urban health and prepare for a future when maintaining a healthy urban environment will be of utmost importance. Also, I hope that this work will inform students about critical urban health issues and, perhaps, inspire some to pursue careers in medicine, the health sciences, and social services, particularly to help those city residents who are underserved and in greatest need.

Acknowledgments

A number of experts in the field of urban health took time from their busy schedules to prepare commentaries on current issues, and their willingness to contribute their professional insight to this work is greatly appreciated. In addition, three health professionals—Alisha Newton, Marilyn Holt, and Yoko Crume—helped research and compile information, providing valuable assistance in keeping the project moving forward. ABC-CLIO's Maxine Taylor offered inestimable guidance and editorial support all along the way, without which this comprehensive and timely treatise on urban health would not have been possible. Many thanks to all of you!

Introduction

Throughout the history of human civilization, most people have lived in rural settings, and it was not until the early twentieth century that large urban areas with populations exceeding 1 million became more commonplace. A milestone was achieved in 2008 when, for the first time, the world's population was evenly divided between urban and nonurban areas, and by the middle of this century, over two-thirds of the world's population will be urban. This represents a remarkable turnabout in human civilization from the early 1800s, when only a small percentage of the world's population lived in cities. Because urban areas present a unique set of circumstances regarding human health, and because urban population growth at the expense of rural areas is expected to continue for the foreseeable future, the need to understand and anticipate urban health issues is becoming more urgent.

Urbanization—the movement of people from rural areas to cities—is one of the twenty-first century's "most transformative trends," according to the New Urban Agenda recently adopted by the United Nations (UN) General Assembly. As global economic activities, social and cultural interactions, and environmental and humanitarian impacts become increasingly concentrated in urban areas, the United Nations believes that the world must prepare for massive sustainability challenges involving human health and other critical urban priorities. In particular, it is concerned that "multiple forms of poverty, growing inequalities, and environmental degradation remain among the major obstacles to sustainability worldwide." As urbanization accelerates over the next few decades, urban health will become inextricably intertwined with the issues surrounding poverty, inequality, and environmental pollution.

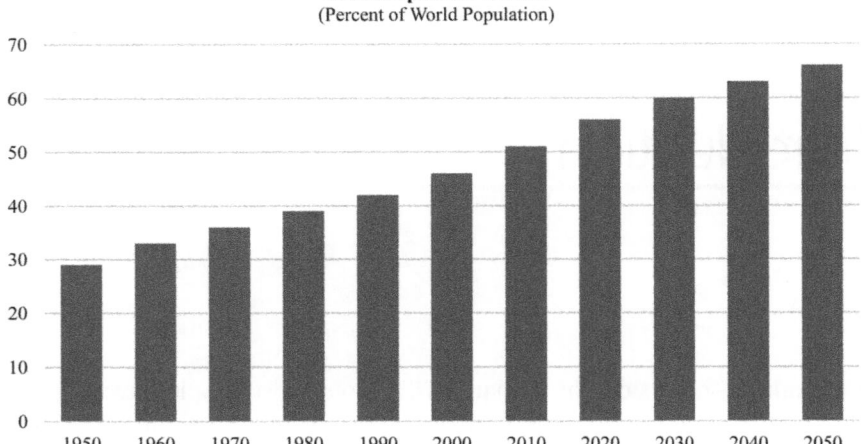

Figure I.1   World Health Organization (2020–2050, based on population projections)

Urban population growth in the twenty-first century will occur most rapidly in developing nations, with people relocating from rural areas to escape poverty and achieve a higher standard of living. This migration from rural to urban areas will become more pronounced by midcentury, as climate change subjects farmlands to more frequent and severe droughts and causes coastal villages to be inundated by rising seawater. Unfortunately, in many of the largest metropolitan areas in the developing world, migrants from the rural countryside end up living in slum areas, where infectious diseases and other serious health problems are rampant. About one-third of the world's urban population lives in slums and informal settlements, often without access to adequate housing, sanitation, and city services. In some cities in developing nations, the slum population approaches 80 percent.

Attempts to characterize the health of urban dwellers are complicated by differing views about just what an urban area is. For example, whether an area is considered urban may vary from country to country, depending on the number of residents, the population density, or the percent of residents engaged in nonagricultural pursuits. In some countries, a city with a population exceeding 2,500 is considered urban, whereas in other countries, the threshold population may be as high as 20,000. Acknowledging the complexity of determining where a rural area ends and an urban area begins, the U.S. Census Bureau uses a combination of population density and land-use characteristics to draw a boundary around an urban area's developed territory, otherwise known as its "footprint." Areas outside the footprint are considered rural. In the United States, rural areas cover 97 percent of the nation's land area but contain less than 20 percent of the total population.

Regardless of how urban areas are defined, as these areas become more densely populated due to migration and more births than deaths, public health concerns emerge that set these areas apart from rural areas. For example, in urban areas, infectious diseases often spread more quickly, there may be more heat-related diseases, and more people suffer from air, light, and noise pollution and offensive odors. Also, urban dwellers may experience more emotional stress and depression if they work long hours in busy office environments and fight heavy traffic commuting to and from work. On the other hand, urban areas may surpass many rural areas in the availability of high-quality healthcare and social services, social support networks, and cultural amenities that add to the quality of life.

In fast-growing urban areas, particularly in developing countries, healthcare services cannot always keep up with population growth due to limited city resources and competition with other priorities. In some of the world's poorest cities, budgets are stretched to the limit just to provide basic water and sanitation services while fighting the spread of infectious diseases. In these cities, where routine healthcare is often unavailable to many residents, health conditions may go untreated until they are serious enough to warrant emergency treatment at a hospital. Even in wealthy countries like the United States, city health services often compete with urgent infrastructure projects (e.g., deteriorating road and sewer systems) and other city priorities for limited public funds. Inadequate healthcare funding is a common reality of cities around the world.

As urbanization accelerates and urban health issues become more complex, cities are taking a more holistic approach to public health that recognizes the interconnectedness of healthcare with other city priorities, such as housing, urban development, and infrastructure improvement. For example, a program aimed at enhancing public transportation options may benefit public health by reducing air pollution, facilitating trips to medical appointments, and lessening the severity of climate change–enhanced heat waves. Furthermore, mental health may benefit from reduced traffic congestion. Similarly, a program to expand neighborhood health clinics may help fight crime and violence by providing free drug and alcohol abuse counseling, and the clinics may improve worker productivity and student performance in school by providing easy access to vaccinations and medical checkups that prevent illnesses. While the value of a holistic approach to healthcare is well established, interdepartmental infighting and competition for funds sometimes preempt constructive collaboration among city programs and departments, to the detriment of public health.

Increasing urbanization has brought to light a growing disparity in healthcare services between those who are well off and those at the lower end of the economic spectrum. Many cities and countries are attempting to address these disparities through a variety of approaches, including free health clinics, expanded health education programs, and universal health insurance, but large disparities in healthcare access and quality remain throughout most parts of the world. Over the next few decades, urban population growth will fuel demands for expanded health services that many cities may be hard pressed to meet without an increased tax base and the political will to provide quality health services even to those least able to pay. Eventually, the world community will need to embrace healthcare for all as a basic human right or suffer the consequences of countless illnesses and deaths that could have been prevented.

Urban Health—A Historical Perspective

The history of urban health dates to the earliest civilizations, perhaps as far back as Egypt's King Djoser (reigned c.2630–c.2611 BCE), when he and his chief minister, Imhotep (27th century BCE), are credited with building the world's first pyramid at Saqqara. (Saqqara was part of the necropolis of the ancient Egyptian city of Memphis.) Imhotep, a man of many talents—architect, mathematician, astronomer, sculptor, poet, priest, and physician—is thought to have written the Edwin Smith Papyrus, an ancient medical text describing nearly 100 anatomical terms and the treatment of 48 types of injuries. Although the papyrus has been dated to around 1600 BCE, which was well after Imhotep's death, it is believed to be a copy of Imhotep's original work, and it is one of the earliest known writings on medicine, as well as the world's oldest-known surgical document. In an extraordinary departure from common beliefs at the time, Imhotep theorized that the diseases and injuries he observed were naturally occurring and not caused by the gods, spirits, or curses.

The Edwin Smith Papyrus is remarkable, not just for its age and documentation of ancient medical theory, but as a seminal document in the history of scientific inquiry. In James Henry Breasted's forward to his translation of the papyrus (University of Chicago Press), he writes:

> In this document, therefore, we have disclosed to us for the first time the human mind peering into the mysteries of the human body, and recognizing conditions and processes there as due to intelligible physical causes. The facts in each given case of injury are observed,

listed, and marshaled before the mind of the observer, who then makes rational conclusions based on the observed facts. Here then we find the first scientific observer known to us, and in this papyrus we have the earliest known scientific document.

Thus, it may be argued that the papyrus represents the first instance of a human applying the scientific method to explore the unknown and draw rational conclusions, and that Imhotep was the world's first true scientist.

ANCIENT EGYPTIAN CIVILIZATION

Priests in Egyptian towns and villages, often serving as physicians, came to believe that injuries and diseases could be treated with a combination of natural remedies and prayer. And as time progressed, these early Egyptian physicians conceived the channel theory—the belief that illness occurs when channels in the human body (i.e., arteries, veins, and intestines) become blocked. Some historians consider this a major turning point in the history of medicine because it represents a societal transition from spiritual cures to a more scientific approach—in this case, eliminating these blockages with laxatives or other natural cures. The ancient Egyptians eventually became surprisingly adept at basic first aid—setting broken bones, treating burns, stitching wounds, and applying bandages. They could also use simple surgical techniques to treat abscesses and tumors, and they knew how to treat skin, dental, eye, and intestinal problems.

Within Egyptian towns, a primitive form of public health often existed, characterized by an emphasis on cleanliness, although mainly for social and religious reasons rather than health. Also, a water supply was commonly present, along with rudimentary baths and toilets, and people were taught to avoid unclean meat and raw fish. On the other hand, some practices were contrary to good public health. For example, while medicines concocted using animal dung may have contained beneficial medicinal molds and fermented substances, they also likely harbored harmful bacteria.

THE GREEKS AND ROMANS

The fundamental concepts on which modern medicine in the Western world is based may have originated with ancient Greek medicine, which was influenced by the Egyptians. The most important figure in Greek medicine was Hippocrates (c.460–c.377 BCE), who conceived what is known in modern times as the Hippocratic Oath, where physicians and other health professionals affirm their adherence to a strict ethical code. Hippocrates promoted the scientific concept of clinical medicine—the study of patients by direct examination—and established medicine as a distinct professional discipline. He also observed that the contaminated air and water in cities can make people ill, and that food, climate, and occupation are also associated with disease. Hippocrates developed a theory about the body being composed of four humors (blood; phlegm; black bile, also known as melancholy; and yellow bile, also known as choler), and he believed that it was necessary to keep the humors in balance to maintain good health. The concept of maintaining balance among the humors influenced the practice of medicine for 2,000 years, and many scholars believe that this theory may have foreshadowed the direction of thought in the development of modern Western medicine (e.g., consuming a balanced diet or achieving good work-life balance). (Other scholars believe the direction of Western medicine originated much earlier, with Imhotep.)

In addition to Hippocrates, other Greek philosophers made important contributions to the science of medicine. For example, Aristotle (348–322 BCE) and Plato (c.428–c.348 BCE) believed that the body had no use in the afterlife—a concept that made the study of human bodies, including dissection, more palatable to society. And the historian Thucydides (d. c.401 BCE) concluded that prayer was ineffective in curing disease.

In the ancient Greek city-states, people had little awareness of public health. For example, the advantages of public sewage systems were unknown, a constant supply of running water was not a priority, and people often appealed to the gods for their healing powers. However, many Greeks, particularly those who were well-off and educated, practiced a healthy lifestyle that included washing the body, cleaning teeth, eating healthy foods, and staying fit, and doctors believed in applying the principle of moderation to daily activities and habits to remain healthy. The ultimate goal was to keep the four humors in balance.

Significant developments in urban health occurred in the Roman Empire, where society seemed to be more interested in preventing than curing diseases. Valuing the importance of good hygiene, the designers of Roman cities included public baths (some with gymnasiums and massage rooms), as well as toilet and sewer systems, and aqueducts were constructed to bring water to urban areas. Some cities also had hospitals, which were initially built to treat injured soldiers and veterans and later were used by other citizens as well. Herbal medicines and pain killers were available, as were medical toolkits for use on the battlefield. Aware that mosquitoes could cause disease, the Romans drained swampy areas in the vicinity of army barracks. Among the famous Roman physicians was Marcus Terentius Varro (116–27 BCE), who became convinced that diseases were caused by tiny organisms too small to be seen (which we know today as bacteria and viruses), and Galen (129–c.199), an expert on human anatomy, who recognized that the brain controls muscle movement through the spinal cord.

CHINA, INDIA, AND THE ISLAMIC PERIOD

As the history of urban health evolved with ancient civilizations in the West, parallel developments were occurring in Eastern countries, particularly China, over a period of 5,000 years or longer. Practitioners of traditional medicine in Chinese towns and villages believed in a life force, *qi* (also known as *chi*), that flows through the body and is composed of opposing elements, yin and yang, that must be kept in balance to maintain good health. Lifestyle was considered important to maintaining this balance (e.g., exercising, eating well, and getting enough sleep), and treatments included herbal medicines, moxibustion (the burning of herbs on or near the skin), acupuncture, and tai chi (meditative movements practiced as a system of exercises). It is estimated that nearly a quarter of the world's population today relies on traditional Chinese medicine, at least as a first resort, with more modern medical practices originating in the West often turned to for the treatment of serious ailments. Traditional Chinese medicine centers and practitioners can be found in urban areas throughout the world.

Traditional Chinese medicine was influenced by two great philosophers, Confucius (551–479 BCE) and Lao-Tzu (6th century BCE). Confucian philosophy, which focused on inner moral harmony and the need to organize social life to maintain political accord, influenced Chinese medicine by offering a metaphorical way of thinking about the human body. For example, to remain healthy, people must regulate and achieve harmony among all aspects of their lives and bodies in the same way that a king regulates affairs to achieve a peaceful and harmonious kingdom. Taoism, founded by Lao-Tzu, was more concerned with self-development and living in harmony with nature through exercise, meditation, and diet. The Tao, sometimes translated into English as "the way," is a cosmic force that unifies and connects all things in the universe, and by submitting to whatever life brings through the Tao, health and happiness can be attained. Both Confucianism and Taoism strongly influenced the direction of traditional Chinese medicine by offering a philosophical framework for understanding health as it relates to human morality, society, and the cosmos.

Ayurvedic medicine (also called Ayurveda), one of the world's oldest medical practices, originated in India over 3,000 years ago, and it continues to be practiced today (sometimes combined with Western medical practices) in towns and villages throughout much of India and Southeast Asia. Ayurvedic medicine is based on belief in a universal connectedness among all people, their health and bodies, and life forces that are often compared to the four humors of ancient Greek medical practice. Illness results when the balance between mind, body, and spirit is disrupted, and treatments are based on herbal medicines, sometimes combined with other substances, such as minerals and metals. Also, special diets, exercise, massage, and body-cleansing techniques may be prescribed. (The U.S. National Center for Complementary and Integrative Health cautions that some Ayurvedic medicinal products used today "may be harmful, particularly if used improperly or without the direction of a trained practitioner.")

During the early Islamic period, believers prayed to God for healing and recovery from disease. However, some sophisticated medical theories and practices developed later, including surgical procedures performed in city hospitals, where opium was used to put patients to sleep prior to surgery. Well-known Islamic physicians included Al-Razi (865–925), who helped develop the field of experimental medicine, established pediatrics as a separate medical field, wrote about immunology and allergies, and recognized that fever is part of the body's natural defense mechanism. Ibn Sina (980–1037) wrote the Canon of Medicine, considered one of the most influential books in medical history, and Ibn al-Nafi (1213–1288) described pulmonary circulation, the movement of blood between the heart and lungs.

THE MIDDLE AGES AND RENAISSANCE

The Middle Ages are often considered a period of stagnation, characterized by superstition and church doctrine, where illness was punishment from God. Nevertheless, some medical research did take place at monasteries, as monks experimented with treatments formulated from their herb gardens. (Monks and nuns were generally the most educated people of this period.) Later in the Middle Ages, as people coalesced into towns and larger cities, medical treatments became more common, often based on Greek and Roman practices, and surgical skills were refined during frequent battles.

Hospitals began to proliferate during the twelfth century to treat soldiers injured in battle.

The Renaissance witnessed major advances in medicine, at a time when epidemics and pandemics proliferated within the growing urban populations as trade with other nations facilitated the spread of infectious agents. The Black Death, a mid-fourteenth-century pandemic of bubonic plague, is estimated to have killed one-third of Europe's population, with the highest percent of deaths occurring in urban areas. Estimates vary on the number of deaths attributed to the disease, but experts believe that more than half of the population died in some European cities—so many that there were not enough survivors left to bury the dead. The number of plague deaths in Europe ranged from 25 to 50 million, and another 25 million may have died in Asia and Africa. Other outbreaks of plague and other infectious diseases have occurred, but the Black Death appears to have had the most far-reaching consequences for human health and society. During this time, new theories developed about how epidemics may be caused by pathogens outside the body that can spread from person to person, and important discoveries were made regarding the human body, for example, the role of the heart in pumping blood. Leonardo da Vinci (1452–1519) famously contributed to medical science's understanding of the mechanical functions of bones and muscles.

IN THE 18TH AND 19TH CENTURIES

With the Industrial Revolution of the eighteenth and nineteenth centuries came remarkable economic growth and urban expansion, but also the onslaught of diseases like typhus and cholera. Meanwhile, yellow fever and other diseases spread as an increasing number of travelers from distant regions passed through cities on their trade routes. Smog blanketed many cities as people burned wood and coal to heat their homes and run factories. Water pollution was common, leading to the spread of infectious diseases, and eventually sanitary systems were developed to protect drinking water from sewage. Many cities instituted trash-removal programs, including the first landfills, to reduce breeding sites for rats that carry disease. Edward Anthony Jenner (1749–1823) created a vaccination to prevent smallpox (the world's first vaccination of any kind), and John Snow (1813–1858), recognized as the father of modern epidemiology, traced the source of cholera outbreaks in London to contaminated drinking water. Later, John Leal (1858–1914), another pivotal figure in the public health field, performed the first continuous disinfection of a municipal drinking water system using chlorine.

MODERN TIMES

By the twentieth century, rapid advancements in the medical and public health fields greatly enhanced the health of city residents. The developments with the greatest benefits to urban health included improved water and sanitation systems, the discovery of penicillin, widespread vaccination programs, better monitoring and control of epidemics, new medicines and treatments, sophisticated diagnostic equipment, state-of-the-art clinics and hospitals, environmental pollution regulations, and antismoking publicity campaigns and ordnances. A new field of public health emerged later in the twentieth century—*environmental health*, defined by the American Public Health Association as "the branch of public health that: focuses on the relationships between people and their environment; promotes human health and well-being; and fosters healthy and safe communities." Among the events leading to the recognition of this new field were a number of catastrophes affecting the health of urban dwellers, including:

- A deadly smog occurring in 1948 in the steel and zinc mining town of Donora, Pennsylvania, that killed 20 people, sickened many more, and led to greater public awareness about air pollution and the need for clean air legislation
- The death of about 4,500 people in 1952 during an unusually severe London smog event, followed by many more deaths in subsequent weeks as the sooty smoke persisted
- A 1956 investigation of neurological symptoms experienced by residents of Minamata, Japan, leading to the discovery of what came be known as "Minamata disease," a form of severe mercury poisoning caused by eating fish and shellfish contaminated by methylmercury in factory wastewater
- Pollution in the Cuyahoga River, running through Cleveland, Ohio, that was so bad that the river caught fire at least a dozen times, including a 1969 incident that grabbed the public's attention
- A 1976 explosion at a chemical plant in Seveso, Italy, releasing a cloud of toxic dioxin gas that descended on the city and other nearby towns, sickening local residents, killing several thousand farm animals, and

causing the slaughter of thousands more farm animals to keep the dioxin out of the food chain

- An accident at the Union Carbide pesticide plant in Bhopal, India, in 1983, resulting in the release of deadly methyl isocyanate and other toxic gases, possibly exposing over 600,000 people to the poisonous gases and killing 15,000 by some estimates

More recently, an environmental disaster struck Fukushima, Japan, and surrounding areas in 2011, when a massive earthquake spawned a 50-foot (15-meter)-tall tsunami that killed around 20,000 people and unleashed a radioactive cloud from the severely damaged Fukushima Daiichi nuclear plant. And in Flint, Michigan, children and other residents were exposed to high lead concentrations in drinking water when city officials switched the water supply to the Flint River in 2014 without implementing proper anticorrosion measures to prevent the release of lead from older water pipes. In some homes, drinking water lead concentrations were ten times higher than the safe level established by the U.S. Environmental Protection Agency (EPA).

The newest threat to environmental health—climate change—will cause stronger and longer droughts, more intense storms and heat waves, the spread of infectious diseases, worse air pollution episodes, food shortages, and eventually, the mass migration of people to more inhabitable areas. Climate change represents a serious threat to urban dwellers, particularly by making heat waves and air pollution more severe and by facilitating the transmission of infectious diseases. Concern over infectious diseases in urban areas is growing, and the World Health Organization (WHO) recently issued the following statement: "Today, worldwide, there is an apparent increase in many infectious diseases, including some newly-circulating ones (HIV/AIDS, hantavirus, hepatitis C, SARS, etc.). This reflects the combined impacts of rapid demographic, environmental, social, technological, and other changes in our ways-of-living. Climate change will also affect infectious disease occurrence."

TODAY'S CHALLENGES

Today, urban health is beset by a bewildering number of challenges— inner-city poverty, drug and alcohol abuse, HIV/AIDS, childhood asthma, environmental degradation, smoking-related illnesses, high cancer rates among both men and women, attention-deficit/hyperactivity disorder among school-age children and young adults, obesity among all age groups, and unacceptable levels of mental illness and suicide, especially among teens and young adults, older adults, and veterans. In developing countries, the spread of infectious diseases in urban areas remains a serious issue, often associated with contaminated water supplies, unsanitary sewage systems, and limited access to quality healthcare for the poorest residents. According to the WHO, there are 4.2 million deaths every year from air pollution, mainly in the large urban areas of developing countries, and another 3.8 million people die annually from indoor pollution caused by household exposure to smoke from dirty cook stoves and fuels.

While the scale of these problems may seem insurmountable, hope lies in (1) the fast pace of innovations in the medical field; (2) standard-of-living improvements in many parts of the world; (3) improved and expanded lifestyle education (e.g., the importance of diet and exercise and the hazards of smoking); and (4) increasing demands within democratic nations for high-quality healthcare for all, regardless of economic and social status. If the history of urban health teaches us anything, it is that seemingly unconquerable health challenges are eventually overcome and that medical science marches on.

Aging and Age-Friendly Communities

Aging is a lifelong biological process that begins at birth, but when people talk about "aging," they generally are referring to a person getting old and beginning to experience functional decline and health problems. In many communities, there is a strong interest in helping older adults live independently, remaining in their homes as long as possible despite their declining functions and health. Furthermore, an increasing number of cities around the world have included the promotion of older adult health and well-being among their highest priorities.

Aging statistics often focus on the population age 65 and older, although there is no specific scientific reasoning behind this age range. In the United States, this practice most likely originated with the Social Security Act of 1935, which set the eligibility age for receiving payments from the Social Security fund at 65 years old. The Social Security Administration explains that this age reflected the common perception of old age in 1935, consistent with the pioneering German pension program, which also set an eligibility age of 65. (Germany was the first nation, in 1889, to establish a social insurance program for older adults.) Today, the retirement age for full benefits gradually increases until it reaches 67 for Americans born after 1959. In contrast, many public health programs in the United States and elsewhere include people age 50 and even younger in their older adult programs, focusing on the prevention of health problems in later years. Nevertheless, age 65 is still used widely in defining old age for statistical purposes.

The most important factor behind the increasing interest in aging and the health of older adults is the remarkable extension of average life expectancy worldwide since the end of World War II. In the half-century between 1950 and 2000, the global average life expectancy increased by 20 years, and by 2050, life expectancy is projected to be 75 years old. In several countries like Japan, where 27 percent of the population is already age 65 or older, an average life expectancy as high as 90 years old may be witnessed even before 2050. As more people live longer, the proportion of older adults in the entire population will also increase, a phenomenon commonly referred to as the "aging society" or "population aging."

Many older adults live in urban areas to be near their working children, to have good healthcare options, and to take advantage of public transportation (for those who do not want to drive or no longer can). Older adults with time on their hands represent a valuable resource for volunteer and community-service work in the city, but they also place increased demands on the healthcare system as they grow older and require more medical attention. Cities often sponsor older adult centers and senior recreation, dining, and transportation programs, but many still struggle to provide the services needed by their expanding older adult population. Notably, because of declining fertility in many developed nations combined with the increasing number of older adults, there are fewer working-age people available to support aging adults, whether by paying taxes, taking care of older parents at home, or supporting aging programs in their communities. This puts an additional strain on city resources.

IMPACT ON URBAN HEALTH

Aging is fundamentally a biological process. As one ages, a wide variety of molecular and cellular changes accumulate, causing a gradual decrease in physiological strength, an increase in the risk of disease, and a decline in overall daily functioning. These conditions become symptomatic for many older adults, although there is more variation in health status among the older adult population than any other age group. While the disease profiles and health conditions of older adults differ somewhat among countries and regions of the world, the older population everywhere is at higher risk of being significantly affected by diseases and functional issues. Furthermore, because many older adults have limited financial resources and fewer family members to lend support, they depend more on city health and social services departments, public wellness programs, and hospital emergency rooms.

About 80 percent of older Americans have at least one, and often two or more, chronic diseases. The most common chronic diseases among older adults are heart disease, cancer, stroke, diabetes, and arthritis. The most common age-related functional declines involve vision and hearing loss, which can greatly affect the quality of life and are closely associated with mental health problems, such as depression and suicide. Moreover, dementia affects an estimated 50 million people worldwide, and most of them are older adults. Physiological changes and functional declines put older adults at higher risk of falling, sometimes resulting in fractures and traumatic brain injuries. Hip fractures can be particularly debilitating, and about 25 percent of older adults sustaining such injuries remain in nursing facilities for at least one year.

A concern for many older adults living in the city, especially those already experiencing health challenges or over 75 years old, is the presence of environmental threats. Along with young children, older adults are especially vulnerable to heat waves, cold spells, air pollution, and communicable diseases, and these threats are often intensified in urban areas, where multiple exposures may be present and diseases can spread through close contact with other residents. During a severe heat wave in Chicago in 1995, 739 deaths were directly linked to the heat, and most of those victims were older adults. Although agencies distributed fans to older residents and cooling centers were available in many neighborhoods, a large number of older adults still suffered. Many lived in low-income apartments without air conditioning, and some were afraid to open their windows for fear of crime. Still others were reluctant to reach out for help, not wanting to be seen as elderly and a burden to society. This illustrates the importance of updating societal attitudes about older adults and being more proactive about addressing their needs so that they feel they are valued members of the community.

Social isolation after retirement is also gaining attention as an important factor affecting the health and well-being of older adults in the city. Some studies have linked social isolation to increased chronic diseases and premature death, and retirement has also been associated with deteriorating health. (Although statistics show improved health during the early years of retirement, the decreasing social contact and activities experienced by many retired people eventually contribute to poorer health.) It is surprising that in a big city surrounded by people, older adults would often suffer from social isolation and loneliness, but a number of studies have found this to be the case. In Tokyo, a major metropolitan area with probably the world's highest proportion of older adults of any big city, the term *kodokushi* (isolation death) is used to describe many instances where socially isolated older adults have been found dead by neighbors, sometimes days or weeks after the death occurred.

In addition to the real health risks associated with older adulthood, the negative perceptions about aging can present serious problems. The term "ageism" was coined in the late 1960s to describe the prevalent age-based stereotyping, prejudice, and discrimination against older people. Since then, efforts have been made to develop a more balanced view toward aging by reframing it as a complex process that is both rewarding and challenging for individuals and society. Reflecting these efforts, the language used to describe older adulthood is also changing. Today, adjectives with negative connotations, such as "senile," "feeble," and "burdensome," are being replaced with positive words, like "active," "productive," and "successful," as a way to confirm the value of older adults to the local communities where they live.

WHAT CITIES ARE DOING ABOUT AGING AND AGE-FRIENDLY COMMUNITIES

Many cities around the world recognize that population aging is a major challenge to their budgets, infrastructures, and resources (or will be soon), and some cities are seeking bold and innovative approaches that go beyond programs offered by their national governments. The mayors of most major U.S. cities have established aging task forces, committees, or other initiatives to identify the needs of their older residents and mobilize city resources to meet those needs. Specifically, these cities commonly focus on (1) providing easy access to health and support services, (2) promoting wellness and disease prevention, (3) creating educational and motivational programs for a healthy lifestyle, and (4) developing age-friendly buildings, sidewalks, and other infrastructure. Often, the federal government provides funding and technical assistance for these types of programs.

American cities are also strengthening ties with other cities around the world to learn directly from their experiences and exchange information on successful aging programs and facilities. Much of this outreach is coordinated by the Global Age-Friendly Cities Project, a project launched by the World Health Organization (WHO) based on the concept that by making cities and communities more age-friendly for everyone, the health and well-being of older people benefit too. The project has published a comprehensive guidebook for developing an age-friendly city, and it offers access to an extensive database of guides, tools, and age-friendly practices. Currently, more than 1,000 cities and communities from 20 nations have signed onto the project. To promote this and other programs, the WHO has identified the following four principles that are important for transforming a city into an age-friendly place to live:

- Recognizing the great diversity among older people
- Promoting their inclusion in all areas of community life
- Respecting their decisions and lifestyle choices
- Anticipating and responding flexibly to aging-related needs and preferences

In the United States, there are many success stories about cities and their aging programs. For example, Iowa City, Iowa, has become one of the best cities for easy healthcare access for older adults because it has been paying close attention to the availability of doctors and clinics and the affordability of their services. In particular, the city enjoys a high ratio of primary-care physicians and dentists to residents, including many specialists in areas of concern to older residents. Healthcare affordability in the city is backed by the state's multifaceted healthcare policies, based on expanded Medicaid services and other federal-, state-, and community-funded programs. Iowa has been rated the most affordable healthcare state, with the lowest percentage of adults who go without adequate healthcare due to inability to pay.

San Francisco, another success story, has been highly effective in promoting disease prevention and management among older adults and others living with chronic conditions, such as arthritis, asthma, diabetes, high blood pressure, and heart disease, by implementing the Chronic Disease Self-Management Program, developed by the Stanford Patient Education Research Center. This program teaches people to manage their health conditions while decreasing stress, fatigue, frustration, and pain, and these services are offered free to all residents, in multiple languages and at many locations throughout the city.

A final example of a success story in an American city is Portland, Oregon, where the city's transportation program exemplifies how an urban area can ensure the mobility of all of its residents, regardless of their disabilities and economic status. The city's extensive transportation network, consisting of buses, light rail trains, streetcars, and even an aerial tram, is considered one of the best in the United States. Additionally, the city implemented an innovative ride-connection program that consolidates an array of agency and nonprofit transportation services into a single entity and links these services to the urban transit system. The vision behind this ride connection initiative was to offer older and disabled residents more adaptable and accessible transportation options while reducing costs through volunteer-based services.

Outside the United States, Berlin is aiming for 100 percent accessibility to businesses and services by widening pavements, adding tactile guidance for visually impaired residents, and improving access to trams and buses. In London, charitable housing for pensioners has been updated with a lounge that opens directly onto the street, where residents can hold craft fairs and bake sales, and even perform plays. Toyama, Japan, promotes easy access to businesses and city services by focusing development around tramway hubs and creating public spaces where people can meet and socialize. In fact, almost every big city in a developed nation has unique initiatives underway to support the older population. Unfortunately, the same cannot be said for low- to middle-income countries, especially in sub-Saharan Africa, where population growth is rapid and often poorly planned and where age-friendly approaches have not yet been embraced.

RECOMMENDATIONS FOR CITY DWELLERS

What is good for the older population is generally also good for younger people. Therefore, aging initiatives can benefit everyone living in the city. People can help make the urban environment age-friendly by embracing universal design elements like no-step entrances, single-floor living, wide halls and doorways, and light-colored indoor surfaces. Also, urban dwellers can work with their building managers and neighbors to ensure that the outdoor environment is safe and walkable so that older adults have an easier time maintaining an active lifestyle, and residents can help prevent social isolation by getting to know their older neighbors and dropping by to check on them now and then.

For older adults living in the city, the single most important step that they can take is to maintain their physical and mental health for as long as possible by exercising regularly, having good nutrition and regular checkups, actively participating in social and community activities, and avoiding drug and alcohol abuse and other destructive behavior. The major health risks to be avoided, due to their strong association with poor health in later years, include tobacco use, physical inactivity, obesity, midlife hypertension, and inadequate calcium intake (which endangers bone health). The good news is that there is increasing evidence that older adults can add years to their lives by making smart choices about diet and lifestyle when younger and then continuing those choices throughout their lifetime.

Air Quality and Urban Smog

Having clean air to breathe is essential to maintaining good health. Yet we often take air quality for granted, perhaps because air pollution is usually invisible, except on days when the pollution is particularly bad. Although we may not always be aware of polluted air, it can affect our health by causing burning eyes, an irritated throat, coughing, and breathing difficulties. Air pollution also increases the risk for acute respiratory infection, and long-term exposure has been associated with cardiovascular disease, stroke, chronic obstructive pulmonary disease (COPD), and lung cancer. During air pollution episodes in large cities, emergency room admissions increase and excess deaths are often recorded, especially when elevated air pollution levels are combined with summertime heat waves.

Many people are surprised to learn that by some measures, air pollution represents the world's greatest single environmental health risk. The World Health Organization (WHO) reports that about 91 percent of the world's population lives in areas where air pollution levels exceed the organization's guideline limits set to protect public health. Approximately 4.2 million premature deaths occur worldwide every year due to exposure to outdoor air pollution, and an additional 3.8 million deaths are due to indoor air pollution. (See the "Indoor Air Quality" entry to learn about air pollution inside buildings.)

Air pollution is widespread across both urban and rural areas, and it can even be found in national parks and nature preserves. However, the highest concentrations usually occur in large urban areas, particularly in low- and middle-income countries, where there is a confluence of industrial and commercial businesses and motor vehicle traffic. Some of the worst air pollution occurs in China and India, where a combined 2 million or more premature deaths may occur annually from outdoor air pollution that is so bad it sometimes obscures the sun at midday, requiring automobiles to burn their headlights at noon.

Although air pollution is a serious global health concern, it is hardly a major component of the air we breathe. In fact, 99 percent of the atmosphere consists of just two benign gases: nitrogen, at 78.1 percent, and oxygen, at 20.9 percent (by volume in dry air); and another 0.9 percent is harmless argon gas. That leaves just 0.1 percent for everything else—ammonia, carbon dioxide, carbon monoxide, helium, hydrogen, iodine, krypton, methane, neon, nitrogen dioxide, ozone, xenon, and various pollutants that are often present in only the part per million (ppm) range or less. (Note: 1 ppm is equivalent to 0.0001 percent.) The air also contains water vapor, which can vary from 1 to 5 percent, and particles such as dust, smoke, acid droplets, and pollen. Despite the relatively low concentrations of pollutants in the air we breathe, the health effects associated with air pollution are well documented.

There are many types of air pollutants, but they generally fall into two categories. First, there are the common air pollutants—carbon monoxide, nitrogen dioxide, lead, ozone, particulate matter, and sulfur dioxide—that tend to be widespread in many large urban areas and can cause both immediate and long-term health problems. (These pollutants are called "criteria air pollutants" in the United States.) Second, there are hazardous air pollutants that tend to be more localized and can cause cancer and other serious, life-threatening health effects. (Hazardous air pollutants are also known as "toxic air pollutants," or more simply, "air toxics.") Examples of hazardous air pollutants are asbestos, benzene, dioxin, methylene chloride, perchloroethylene, toluene, and metals such as cadmium, mercury, chromium, and lead compounds. The U.S. Clean Air Act recognizes 188 separate hazardous air pollutants, and there are probably many others, including new chemicals created after the most recent Clean Air Act amendments.

Among the six common air pollutants, the two of greatest concern today in urban areas are ozone and particular matter (PM). In contrast to most other forms of air pollution, ozone is not emitted directly into the air. Instead, it is formed near ground level when nitrogen oxides (mixtures of highly reactive gases containing nitrogen and oxygen) and volatile organic compounds (carbon-containing compounds that participate in atmospheric photochemistry) react in the presence of sunlight, especially on warm summer days. (The ground-level ozone discussed here should not be confused with the "good" ozone that occurs naturally in the stratosphere, some 31 miles, or 50 kilometers, above the earth's surface, helping shield the earth from harmful ultraviolet radiation from the sun.) Smog, a type of air pollution that is common in many metropolitan areas, consists primarily of ozone and a mixture of several other air pollutants, such as carbon monoxide, nitrogen oxides, sulfur dioxide, small particles, and volatile organic compounds.

Like ozone, PM is a widespread problem in many urban areas, especially for children, older adults, and people with existing heart or lung disease. PM is a complex mixture of particles and liquid droplets of many sizes. Most PM that is small enough to enter the lungs results from chemical reactions in the atmosphere involving organic compounds and gases such as sulfur dioxide and nitrogen oxides, and some small PM also originates with forest and structure fires and dust from unpaved roads and construction sites. PM with a diameter of 10 micrometers and smaller (often written as PM_{10}) is of particular concern because it can be inhaled directly into the lungs without being captured by the throat and nose, and fine PM, having a diameter of 2.5 micrometers and less (often written as $PM_{2.5}$), can reach the most remote regions of the lungs.

Lead, one of the listed common air pollutants, is not the concern it once was in the United States, where lead concentrations in the ambient air have been reduced by 98 percent as a result of regulations removing lead from gasoline. Nevertheless, industrial sources of lead air pollution remain in some areas, and serious lead exposures still occur from lead in drinking water caused by the corrosion of plumbing materials and from lead-based paint in older homes. Soils near industrial sites can also be contaminated with lead.

Lead air pollution is much more of a problem in low- and middle-income countries, where emissions may occur during smelting, recycling, and other industrial operations, and where it may still be used in gasoline and aviation fuel. The WHO reports that lead exposure from all sources may have accounted for about 500,000 deaths and 12 percent of the global burden of idiopathic developmental intellectual disability in 2015.

Carbon dioxide (CO_2) is another type of air pollutant, although some scientists debate whether it should be labeled "air pollution" because CO_2 is naturally present in the atmosphere as part of the earth's carbon cycle, and it does not adversely affect human health by itself. However, there is grave concern among scientists about climate change caused by increasing atmospheric concentrations of CO_2 and other greenhouse gases (GHGs) associated with human activities, particularly the combustion of fossil fuels to generate electricity. (See the "Climate Change" entry to learn more about CO_2.)

The air pollution found in urban areas comes from a variety of sources. These include motor vehicles, electric power plants that burn fossil fuels, oil and gas refineries, plastics and chemical manufacturing companies, cement and asphalt plants, and a large variety of smaller commercial businesses. Additionally, there are natural sources of air pollution, like the gases and particles coming from volcanos and forest fires and the wind-blown dust common in many arid areas of the world.

Air pollution sources are classified in different ways. For example, cars, trucks, buses, trains, and airplanes are called "mobile sources," whereas most industrial and commercial operations are called "stationary sources." Stationary sources are further broken into two categories: "point sources," where the pollution is emitted from a specific point like a smokestack; and "area sources," where the pollution emanates from a large number of smaller sources, such as dry cleaners, automobile repair and body shops, gas stations, fast food restaurants, and small incinerators. Individually, an area source may not emit much air pollution, but when all the area sources in a city are taken together, the aggregate air pollution can be substantial. For this reason, area sources, along with mobile sources and stationary sources, are major concerns in urban areas.

IMPACT ON URBAN HEALTH

How city residents react to air pollution depends not only on the type of air pollutant, but also on the concentration of the pollutant in the air, the duration of exposure, and whether other pollutants are present that cause synergistic effects. Elevated temperature and humidity can also add to the discomfort and worsen any symptoms that exist. When heat waves in urban areas combine with high air pollution levels, the results can be deadly.

An individual's susceptibility to air pollution is also important in understanding effects on health. For example, someone with asthma, a compromised immune system, or some other preexisting health condition may be more likely to exhibit health effects from air pollution exposure. Children and older adults are particularly vulnerable to air pollution, and some people are simply more sensitive to air pollution, regardless of age.

Breathing ozone, the main component of urban smog, can cause a variety of adverse health effects. In particular, it can irritate the respiratory system, elicit chest pain, aggravate asthma, and reduce overall lung function. Ozone can also inflame and even damage the linings of the lungs, similar to sunburn on exposed skin, and it can quickly trigger respiratory discomfort and distress in children, older adults, and people with lung diseases like asthma. In addition to threatening health, ozone can harm sensitive vegetation in urban gardens and landscaping, especially during the growing season.

Similar to ozone, the PM air pollution common in urban areas has been associated with a number of adverse health effects. This is especially true for the smallest particles, which can penetrate to the lowest reaches of the lungs. Many scientific studies have linked PM to premature death in people with heart or lung disease, nonfatal heart attacks, and irregular heartbeat. Additionally, PM is associated with aggravated asthma, decreased lung function, and increased respiratory symptoms, such as irritation of the airways, coughing, and difficulty breathing; and a recent study found a significant association between fine particulate air pollution and the risk of diabetes.

The other four common air pollutants—carbon monoxide, lead, nitrogen dioxide, and sulfur dioxide—can also cause health problems. Exposure to carbon monoxide reduces oxygen delivery to the heart, brain, and other tissues, and extremely high levels can cause death. Lead air pollution can affect kidney function and the nervous, immune, reproductive, developmental, and cardiovascular systems. Also, lead diminishes the oxygen-carrying capacity of the blood, and it can cause behavioral problems and lower IQ in infants and young children. Nitrogen dioxide can cause respiratory problems and contribute to ground-level ozone and fine PM formation; similarly, sulfur dioxide can cause respiratory problems and contributes to the formation of fine PM.

Hazardous air pollutants represent a different type of problem in urban areas for three reasons: (1) they are often localized around specific sources; (2) the health effects associated with hazardous air pollutants may occur at very low concentrations in the atmosphere; and (3) certain serious health conditions associated with hazardous air pollutants, such as cancer, may take years to develop. Other serious health conditions can include damage to the immune system and various neurological, reproductive, developmental, and respiratory problems. Additionally, hazardous air pollutants can harm the environment and degrade our food supply, such as when mercury is magnified through the food chain. (Fish and shellfish are particularly susceptible.) Exposure to hazardous air pollutants usually occurs by breathing contaminated air. However, exposure can also occur when eating foods and drinking water that have come into contact with contaminated air, and young children can be exposed through ingestion or skin contact when playing in soil, dust, or water contaminated by hazardous air pollution. Low-income and minority groups living close to industrial and commercial areas and major roadways are sometimes disproportionately exposed to hazardous air pollutants. (This means that their exposure is higher than other people having the means to live in cleaner parts of the city or suburbs.)

Children living in the city are particularly at risk from air pollution because their lungs are still developing and they breathe more air on a body-weight basis than adults. Also, children tend to spend more time outdoors in the polluted air, and many children suffer from asthma, which is aggravated by air pollution. Many older adults, especially those with lung disease, are also sensitive to poor air quality. For example, ozone and PM can aggravate asthma, COPD, and other health conditions affecting older adults, leading to hospitalization and even premature death. Adults generally become more sensitive to air pollution in their mid-sixties, although the risk of heart attack associated with particle pollution may begin as early as the mid-fifties for women and mid-forties for men. In addition to children and older adults, pregnant women and people with existing medical conditions may experience enhanced sensitivity to polluted air.

WHAT CITIES ARE DOING ABOUT AIR POLLUTION

Many industrialized countries have made great strides in reducing air pollution emissions, but serious problems remain. In the United States, air pollution emissions of the six common pollutants declined by 73 percent between 1970 (when the Clean Air Act was enacted) and 2017. This is a significant accomplishment, given that other factors that would tend to increase pollution have increased over the same time frame—for instance, energy consumption increased 44 percent, population 59 percent, vehicle miles traveled 189 percent, and gross domestic product 262 percent. Nevertheless, in 2017, there were still over 110 million Americans living in parts of the country—mainly large urban areas—that experience air pollution levels exceeding national ambient air quality standards. Similarly, despite tough air pollution regulations in many other countries, a large numbers of urban dwellers throughout the world continue to experience unacceptably high levels of air pollution.

Motor vehicles often contribute more to urban air pollution than any other sources. Automobile emissions are about 99 percent cleaner than they were back in the 1970s because of technological innovations, such as the catalytic converter, computerized controls, fuel injection, and on-board diagnostics. (Some scientists regard the catalytic converter as one of the greatest environmental inventions of all time.) Even so, because of the large number of motor vehicles on the road (an estimated 250 million in the United States and 1 billion or more worldwide), vehicles contribute vast amounts of urban air pollution.

To reduce motor vehicle emissions, cities have taken a wide variety of steps, including the following:

- Incorporating tailpipe emission testing into automobile registration and renewal requirements
- Synchronizing traffic lights to reduce starts and stops at intersections
- Encouraging use of public transportation, ride-sharing, carpooling, and high-occupancy vehicle lanes
- Creating bicycle lanes and improving sidewalks
- Restricting automobile use at certain times of the day, on specific days of the week, or in central locations, like the city core
- Purchasing low-emission buses and garbage trucks powered by electricity or natural gas
- Promoting hybrid- and electric-vehicle use by providing charging stations and dedicated parking spots
- Collecting a fee for driving in the city core
- Banning older vehicles on city streets

Air pollution emissions from diesel trucks are a particular problem in many urban areas that experience heavy truck traffic, and cities have taken various steps to address this source of pollution, including providing financial assistance to replace older trucks with newer models that pollute less. Other successful approaches to reduce truck air pollution emissions include installing retrofit technology to improve engine performance, reducing truck idling time, performing regular engine maintenance, tracking fuel consumption and other engine performance parameters, providing driver training, and installing low-rolling resistance tires, automatic tire inflation systems, and truck aerodynamic features. Diesel-truck fleet owners will often take these steps voluntarily, especially if financial assistance and other incentives are available, because of the cost savings associated with reduced fuel consumption. To reduce air pollution and become carbon neutral, several countries are planning to ban future diesel automobile sales.

To protect urban residents from unacceptably high levels of air pollution from industrial and commercial facilities, city officials ensure that permits to build and operate these facilities demonstrate compliance with any federal air pollution regulations. In the United States, this means compliance with air pollution emission regulations that have been developed for a large number of industries and commercial operations. (Additionally, the states must show that air quality will not exceed limits established in national ambient air quality standards.) Cities and states can also set their own air pollution regulations, and often permits to build and operate facilities will not be granted if doing so would cause a city, state, or federal regulation to be violated. Most developed countries take a similar approach, although air pollution regulations in the United States are among the world's toughest and often serve as models for other nations.

To comply with air pollution regulations, an industrial or commercial facility may need to modify its operations or install air pollution control equipment. These steps can be very expensive, and in extreme cases, the company may close a facility or locate a new facility elsewhere rather than incurring these costs. However, the benefits to urban health from air pollution regulations—fewer illnesses, a smaller number of missed days from work and school, greater work productivity, and lower medical and insurance costs—far outweigh the costs to develop, implement, and comply with air pollution regulations, according to most experts.

In addition to enforcing air pollution regulations, cities can ban certain types of facilities, like incinerators; require other facilities to be located away from residential areas; and mandate that existing facilities retrofit pollution control technologies. Cities can also limit wood-burning residential stoves and heaters, ban outdoor burning of yard trimmings and other plant debris, and encourage the use of clean, renewable energy. To reduce emissions from electric power plants, many cities and utility companies offer assistance with insulating and weather-stripping homes to prevent heat loss during the winter and air conditioning loss in the summer. These measures aimed at cutting energy use have the added benefit of reducing residential heating and air conditioning bills.

Another strategy employed by cities to reduce air pollution is to plant trees and other greenery, which help keep the city cool and reduce air conditioning demand. With less air conditioning, energy consumption is reduced, resulting in less air pollution from power plants. Also, lower temperatures help reduce smog formation. City temperatures can also be reduced by replacing dense materials like concrete and asphalt pavement with green spaces, which helps to reduce the urban heat island effect (i.e., higher city temperatures caused by the abundance of dense, heat-absorbing construction and road materials). (For more information on the heat island effect, see the "Climate Change" and "Green Buildings and Sustainable Development" entries to learn more about the heat island effect.)

RECOMMENDATIONS FOR CITY DWELLERS

Because the average person breathes over 3,000 gallons (11.4 cubic meters) of air each day, there is a good chance that any air pollutants in the surrounding air will find their way into the lungs and bloodstream. (Air pollution can also be absorbed through the skin.) Thus, urban dwellers need to be careful to limit their time in polluted areas (or avoid them altogether), and to stay indoors on days when the air quality is poor. Also, people should avoid areas in the city where air pollution tends to be greatest—along busy roadways, near industrial and commercial operations that emit air pollutants, and within areas where air pollution may concentrate, like busy parking garages. Burning eyes, throat irritation, coughing, and shortness of breath may be signs that the surrounding air is heavily polluted.

A number of countries have air pollution warning systems that alert citizens to the potential for poor air quality, and many of these programs are modeled after the AirNow air quality alert system developed by the U.S. Environmental Protection Agency (EPA). The principal service offered by AirNow is the Air Quality Index (AQI), which provides air quality information to the public using a numerical and color-coded scale. (The AQI is concerned with air pollution exposure over a few hours or days, and it does not predict health effects from exposure over longer periods.) The AQI ranks air quality from 0 to 500, as illustrated in Table 1. As the index number gets higher, the potential health concerns become more severe and affect more people. For example, a value of 50 (color coded green) indicates good air quality, while a value over 300 (color coded maroon) represents hazardous air quality. Generally, values above 100 are considered unhealthy

Table 1   AQI Range, Color, and Level of Health Concern

Range	Color Code	Level of Health Concern
0–50	Green	**Good**—Air quality is satisfactory and poses little or no health risk.
51–100	Yellow	**Moderate**—Air quality is acceptable; however, pollution in this range may pose a moderate health concern for a very small number of individuals. People who are unusually sensitive to ozone or particle pollution may experience respiratory symptoms.
101–150	Orange	**Unhealthy for Sensitive Groups**—Although the general public is not likely to be affected at this AQI range, people with lung disease, older adults, children, and people who are active outdoors are at a greater risk from exposure to ozone; and people with heart and lung disease, older adults, and children are at greater risk from the presence of particles in the air.
151–200	Red	**Unhealthy**—Everyone may begin to experience some adverse health effects, and members of sensitive groups may experience more serious effects.
201–300	Purple	**Very Unhealthy**—AQI levels in this range would trigger a health alert, signifying that everyone may experience more serious health effects.
301–500	Maroon	**Hazardous**—AQI levels in this range would trigger health warnings of emergency conditions. The entire population is even more likely to be affected by serious health effects.

Source: EPA.

for sensitive individuals, and almost everyone begins to experience adverse health effects when the AQI exceeds 150. The AQI is reported for five common air pollutants—carbon monoxide, nitrogen dioxide, ozone, PM, and sulfur dioxide.

By making themselves aware of outdoor air quality, people can modify their daily routines, such as staying indoors and limiting exercise, when the

AQI is poor. AQI updates are provided during many local TV weather forecasts, especially when poor air quality is a concern for people spending time out of doors, and the updates are also carried by The Weather Channel and other media outlets. Additionally, the AQI is available on the Internet. AirNow International is an international version of AirNow for use by cities in other countries.

CITY SPOTLIGHT: MEXICO CITY—GRIPPED BY A NAGGING AIR POLLUTION PROBLEM

Once plagued by air pollution so severe that birds fell from the sky, Mexico City has made great progress in reducing toxic gases and cleaning up its air. But much more progress is needed if the city is to realize clean air goals on par with large urban areas in the United States and Europe.

As one of the world's largest metropolises, Mexico City has struggled over the years with high air pollution levels that dim the morning sunlight and compromise the health of its 21 million metropolitan inhabitants. The city is mostly surrounded by mountains, which tend to hold the pollution in place, and the stagnant weather conditions are made worse by high summertime temperatures. Because of the dense and widespread air pollution, Mexico City was once dubbed the world's most polluted city.

Air pollution levels began to fall in the 1990s and 2000s, when some of the most polluting industries moved away and the city implemented programs aimed at improving public transportation, limiting air pollution emissions from factories and vehicles, and more recently, developing a very popular bike-sharing program. (Reduced speed limits were also introduced to cut air pollution emissions from vehicles, although some experts question the effectiveness of this approach.) A program called Hoy No Circula (No Drive Days) prohibited driving one day every week (the specific day based on the car's license plate number), and this program was later expanded to include one Saturday per month (also depending on license plate number). Today, Mexico City is no longer the world's most polluted city, but its air pollution still ranks high among other large metropolitan areas, and in a typical year, there are far more days when the air quality is poor than when it is clean.

An important reason for Mexico City's ongoing air pollution problem is its very large population, which continues to grow as people move to the city for business opportunities and better-paying jobs. Additionally, there have been some cultural barriers to pollution control programs, such as reluctance to use public transportation because owning and driving a car are status symbols and sources of pride for many poor families. Another issue is that people find ways to circumvent the Hoy No Circula program, such as getting someone else to drive them on days when they should not be driving, or buying a second car (often an older, polluting model) to use on those days. And because some car owners pay bribes at vehicle inspection stations, a number of older cars remain on the streets despite their high pollution levels. Dust blowing over the city from nearby deforested terrain also contributes to the air pollution, as do agricultural crop burning to clear fields, fossil fuel combustion for electric power and other industrial purposes, uncontrolled trash burning in open containers or pits, and increasingly longer commutes from the suburbs as newer residents are forced to live farther from the city center.

Looking toward the future, Mexico recently developed tough new emission standards for heavy-duty diesel vehicles, soot-free buses have begun operating in downtown areas of Mexico City, and diesel cars will eventually be banned from the streets. However, most experts caution that these measures alone will not be enough. Ultimately, the city must expand public transportation options and make public transportation more attractive to city residents so that there is less incentive to use personal vehicles. For example, although the subway is cheap and connects many parts of the city, the trains can be incredibly crowded, and women often consider the subway unsafe. (Many people prefer ride-sharing services like Uber, believing it to be a safer and more reliable option.) The city also needs to implement tougher vehicle emission inspections and move more rapidly on other environmental programs, which some observers believe have been delayed by bureaucratic lethargy and corruption.

The air pollution problems facing Mexico City are similar to other large cities in developing countries—population growth, inadequate or unpopular public transportation options, bureaucratic delays, continued reliance on fossil fuels, and cultural factors that encourage car ownership. Time will tell if Mexico City will ever get its air pollution problem under control, but with new regulations and a revived commitment to improving air quality, there is every reason to be optimistic.

Chemical Exposure

Chemicals are all around us, and if we live in the city, we are exposed to chemicals almost all the time. Chemicals are in the air we breathe and the water and food we consume, and we can even be exposed through our skin when we touch contaminated surfaces. Most chemicals are harmless, and some are even good for us (such as the chemicals in medicines). But other chemicals can make us sick, sometimes causing serious illness and even death.

We often think of chemicals as liquids on a laboratory shelf or in a tanker truck that are used in products like plastics and petroleum. However, the definition of the term "chemical" is actually much broader. Simply put, a chemical is an element (i.e., a primary constituent of matter) or a combination of elements that has a specific composition and structure. Thus, a chemical can be as basic as oxygen or water, or it can have a highly complex structure comprising many molecules. Human beings and all other life on Earth, including the foods we eat, are composed of chemicals.

Health professionals are not concerned with chemicals per se, but with *toxic* chemicals—those that can make us sick. When we see a product on the grocery store shelf labeled "chemical free," that is a misnomer because the product itself is made of chemicals. What this statement really means is that the product is free of added chemicals that may harm our health or the environment—in other words, toxic chemicals. The challenge to health and environmental scientists lies in determining what chemicals are toxic and how to reduce or eliminate exposure to these chemicals.

For people living in urban areas, exposure to toxic chemicals can occur inside homes, schools, and businesses, and exposure can also happen outside while going to work, shopping, or exercising in a city park. Indoor sources of chemical exposure may include (1) consumer products and appliances, such as household cleaners, personal care products, indoor pesticides, woodstoves, and fireplaces; (2) building materials, including carpeting, drywall, insulation, and composite wood flooring and furniture; (3) radon gas, which has seeped into the building from soil, rock, and foundation materials; (4) drinking water contaminated with lead or other toxic pollutants; (5) food contaminated with pesticides, mercury, or other unsafe chemicals; and (6) hazardous raw materials and solvents used at some manufacturing facilities. The major source of outdoor exposure to chemicals is the surrounding air when it becomes polluted with toxic gases and particles from motor vehicles, commercial and industrial operations, landfills and other waste management facilities, and power plants. Chemical exposure can also occur at abandoned waste disposal sites when chemicals leak from underground containment vessels, contaminating soil surfaces.

Because chemical use is widespread throughout the world, and because many chemicals are persistent in the environment and do not break down easily, trace amounts of toxic chemicals can be found in the bodies of almost every human. These chemicals include bisphenol A (used in manufacturing polycarbonate plastics and epoxy resins, which have a wide variety of applications, including food packaging); dichloro-diphenyl-trichloroethane (commonly known as DDT), a pesticide now banned in the United States and other countries; perfluorooctanoic acid (used in manufacturing nonstick coatings for cookware); polybrominated diphenyl ethers (flame retardants used in electronic devices, furniture, textiles, and other household products); and polychlorinated biphenyls (a once popular chemical for electrical, heat transfer, and hydraulic equipment that is now banned in the United States and other countries). Although some particularly egregious chemicals like DDT have been banned, chemicals remain ubiquitous in the environment.

IMPACT ON URBAN HEALTH

Because thousands of chemicals are widely used in commerce today (no one knows the exact number), it is difficult to list each one and discuss all the possible health outcomes from exposure. Nevertheless, there are some chemicals that are especially concerning to health professionals due to their known or suspected toxicity to major systems of the human body, as illustrated in Table 2. While living in the city, it would not be unusual to be exposed to many of these and other chemicals on a daily basis, although at

Table 2   Some Chemicals That Can Harm Systems of the Human Body

Human Body System	Chemical (Examples of Sources)
Cardiovascular system	• Carbon disulfide (industrial production) • Carbon monoxide (car exhaust, unvented or faulty furnaces) • Methylene chloride (auto part cleaners, paint removers) • Nitrates (fertilizers)
Hepatic system	• Carbon tetrachloride (adhesives) • Methylene chloride (auto part cleaners, paint removers) • Vinyl chloride (pipe sealer)
Immune system	• Lead (old paint, outdated plumbing) • Mercury (thermostats, thermometers, contaminated fish) • Pesticides (unwashed fruits and vegetables) • Polychlorinated biphenyls (industrial waste, contaminated fish) • Polycyclic aromatic hydrocarbons (cigarette smoke, vehicle exhaust, asphalt roads)
Nervous system	• Arsenic (pressure-treated wood) • Cadmium (discarded batteries, cigarette smoke) • Carbon monoxide (car exhaust, unvented or faulty furnaces) • Cyanide (rat poison)
Renal system	• Cadmium (discarded batteries, cigarette smoke) • Chlorinated hydrocarbon solvents (degreasers, paint removers, dry cleaning solutions) • Lead (old paint, outdated plumbing) • Mercury (thermostats, thermometers, contaminated fish) • Uranium (food and water near nuclear testing sites)

(*continued*)

Table 2   (continued)

Human Body System	Chemical (Examples of Sources)
Reproductive system	• Methyl mercury (contaminated fish, coal-burning power plants) • Carbon monoxide (car exhaust, unvented or faulty furnaces) • Lead (old paint, outdated plumbing)
Respiratory system	• Asbestos (old insulation) • Radon (soil, rock, building foundation materials) • Cadmium (old batteries) • Benzene (degreasers) • Carbon monoxide (car exhaust, unvented or faulty furnaces) • Soot (furnaces, wood-burning stoves)
Skin	• Arsenic (pressure-treated wood) • Chromium (paints, industrial production) • Mercury (thermostats, thermometers, contaminated fish) • Nickel (cement) • Polychlorinated biphenyls (industrial waste, contaminated fish) • Volatile organic compounds (fumes from gasoline, paint, adhesives, building supplies)

Source: Agency for Toxic Substances and Disease Registry.

concentrations too low to be of concern most of the time. Some examples of toxic chemical exposure in the urban environment are the following:

• At home or work, city residents may inhale formaldehyde and other volatile organic compounds given off by building materials and electronic equipment, and they also may be exposed to radon gas that has infiltrated buildings from the soil, rock, and foundation materials below.

- While walking to school or work, particularly along busy city streets, people may be exposed to ozone and to automobile and truck exhausts containing carbon monoxide, nitrogen oxides, volatile organic compounds, and particulates.
- Factory workers could potentially be exposed to a wide variety of chemicals, such as arsenic, benzene, cadmium, carbon disulfide, carbon tetrachloride, chromium, mercury, methylene chloride, nickel, and vinyl chloride.
- While renovating old homes or other buildings in the city, homeowners and contractors risk being exposed to asbestos in wall and ceiling insulation, lead in old paint, and other hazardous substances, and they may not even realize that these materials are present.
- The fish that residents buy at a local market or grocery store might be contaminated with mercury, and the vegetables could contain pesticide residue.
- Sometimes even water can be contaminated, as the residents of Flint, Michigan, recently discovered when symptoms of lead poisoning were traced to lead in drinking water.

The health effects associated with exposures to toxic chemicals can range from minor symptoms, such as headache and fatigue, to serious, debilitating, and even life-threatening conditions, such as injury to the nervous and immune systems, respiratory and cardiovascular diseases, birth defects, and many types of cancer. Children exposed to toxic chemicals may also suffer from developmental problems and learning disabilities. Children, older adults, pregnant women, and people with disabilities or preexisting diseases may be more susceptible to toxic chemical exposure, and health professionals advise taking extra precautions to minimize exposure for these individuals.

The symptoms of exposure to some toxic chemicals will become evident almost immediately, while symptoms for other chemicals may take longer to appear. Toxic chemicals causing cancer (i.e., carcinogens) are ordinarily associated with a long latency period, which means that a number of years may pass before the cancer appears. Thus, exposure to carcinogens during childhood or early adulthood may not become evident until middle age or later. In contrast to many other toxic chemicals, carcinogens may lack a threshold below which no health effects will occur. In other words, toxicologists believe there may be no safe level of exposure for toxic chemicals that cause cancer, although research on this topic continues.

Another characteristic of toxic chemicals is that they may be very persistent in the human body, remaining there for many years or even a lifetime. Furthermore, some may bioaccumulate up the food chain, resulting in higher concentrations for humans consuming certain fish and other wildlife. Some toxic chemicals are endocrine disruptors, which disrupt the hormone system, and others are known to cause reproductive problems and damage deoxyribonucleic acid (DNA), the hereditary material that determines who we are as individuals.

The exposure of young children to toxic chemicals like lead is particularly concerning because children may exhibit greater vulnerable to toxicity as their bodies develop. Childhood exposure to lead can result from lead in domestic water-supply pipes, lead in paint, leaded cans for food and drink, and lead in cosmetics and folk remedies. (Leaded gasoline, once considered a serious public health problem, has been banned in most countries.) Exposure to lead, even at relatively low levels, can cause reduced IQ scores, learning disabilities, poor performance in school, anemia, and violent behavior; and exposure at higher levels can cause serious neurological problems. Another concern for children is exposure to pesticides (i.e., insecticides, herbicides, and rodenticides). Although pesticide exposure is more of a problem in rural agricultural areas, acute pesticide poisoning among toddlers also can occur in cities when young children explore pesticide containers in their homes, garden sheds, or garages.

Can we assume that all chemicals have been tested for safety and that all potential health effects have been identified? Unfortunately, this is not the case. For example, in the United States, among the approximately 2,000 new industrial chemicals introduced each year and the thousands already on the market, toxicological tests have been performed on only a small percentage. The exception is for chemicals produced by pharmaceutical and pesticide companies, which ordinarily undergo extensive testing before marketing.

WHAT CITIES ARE DOING ABOUT CHEMICAL EXPOSURE

Chemical exposure in the city is ordinarily not addressed by a single office or agency, but rather by a number of entities addressing various aspects of the problem and often working together to address complex situations. Some examples of these entities and their roles in reducing chemical exposure are the following:

- **Building permits and inspections office**—Ensures that the design and construction of new buildings and the renovation of existing buildings comply with guidelines for safe materials and good ventilation, thereby helping to minimize toxic chemicals in the indoor air
- **Energy coordinator**—Advises citizens and city government on low-polluting, renewable energy sources and helps develop government energy and environmental policies that reduce toxic chemicals in the outdoor air
- **Environmental pollution control office**—Monitors air and water quality, coordinates the cleanup of waste sites, administers vehicle emissions testing programs, issues public alerts for poor air quality days, and enforces rules, all aimed at reducing toxic chemical pollution and protecting public health
- **Health department**—Investigates disease outbreaks that could be linked to chemical exposure, educates the public on chemical exposure, and conducts restaurant inspections (e.g., to ensure that vegetables are washed to remove any chemical residues)
- **Hospital emergency rooms and urgent care centers**—Treat victims of chemical burns, respiratory distress from smog episodes, carbon monoxide poisoning, and other chemical exposures
- **Office of emergency management**—Coordinates the response to large chemical spills and other emergency situations involving hazardous chemicals
- **Public safety and fire departments**—Often the first responders to serious chemical exposures occurring at home or following vehicle accidents
- **Public works office**—Manages trash collection and recycling programs, including the collection and recycling of household hazardous chemicals like paints, solvents, and fuels
- **Transit authority**—Coordinates with state or regional officials to ensure that bulk chemicals are transported safely within the city
- **Universities**—Conduct research on the health effects of chemical exposure and provide guidance on cleanup and disposal issues
- **Water services office**—Manages drinking water systems, ensuring a clean and healthy water supply free of toxic chemical concentrations that are high enough to affect public health

Not all urban areas provide these services, and some cities may combine services or offer them jointly with other jurisdictions. Also, cities generally do not develop their own chemical regulations (e.g., to limit exposure to air and water pollution, protect workers from toxic chemical exposure, ban hazardous chemicals from consumer products, and regulate interstate transport of hazardous chemicals). Instead, these types of regulations with broad applications to cities and regions tend to be developed at the state, regional, and federal levels of government.

RECOMMENDATIONS FOR CITY DWELLERS

Because city dwellers are surrounded by chemicals in the air, water, building materials, and consumer products, they can never hope to totally eliminate all chemical exposure. However, by following these guidelines, people can manage their exposure and reduce their risk of illness:

- Read the labels on consumer products that warn about toxic ingredients and follow the instructions carefully, or completely avoid these products.
- Learn about and avoid any chemical contamination around homes, schools, industrial areas, construction sites, and hazardous material dump sites.
- Wash hands frequently, and thoroughly wash fruits and vegetables.
- Follow local fish advisories, such as recommendations to avoid fish containing high levels of mercury. (However, many health professionals consider low-mercury fish part of a healthy diet.)
- Be sure that fireplaces and wood-burning stoves are vented to the outside, and never burn wood that has been chemically treated, painted, or varnished.
- Do not keep any longer than necessary products containing toxic chemicals, such as paints, varnishes, pesticides, batteries, and some electronics and cleaning products, and be sure to follow the disposal guidelines provided by your local waste disposal office.
- Ensure that houses and apartments are well ventilated by regularly running the ventilation system or opening windows.
- Never smoke tobacco products, and avoid secondhand and thirdhand smoke. (Thirdhand smoke is defined by the Mayo Clinic as residual nicotine and other chemicals left on indoor surfaces by tobacco smoke.)

City residents may also want to consider purchasing "green" products manufactured using the principles of green chemistry, which involve reducing or eliminating toxic chemicals. These principles apply to the entire life cycle of a product—its design, manufacture, use by the consumer, and ultimate disposal. Green chemistry can lessen exposure to toxic chemicals while reducing air and water pollution and toxic waste disposal in your community. While there is no single way of applying green chemistry, most applications are based on some combination of preventing waste, maximizing the efficient use of materials, reducing or eliminating toxic chemicals from the manufacturing process, increasing energy efficiency, using renewable feedstock, designing chemicals and products to degrade after use, and emphasizing safety and accident reduction or prevention.

People exposed to toxic chemicals do not automatically get sick. A number of factors determine if they will become ill and how serious the illness is, such as (1) the type and amount of chemical they were exposed to; (2) the duration of exposure and how often they were exposed; (3) whether exposure occurred by inhalation, ingestion, or dermal contact; (4) their overall health and ability to fight off any toxic effects; and (5) their sensitivity to toxic chemicals. If you are concerned about chemical exposure, your doctor can diagnose symptoms and prescribe treatments or refer you to a specialist if necessary.

EXPERT COMMENTARY: ENVIRONMENTAL HEALTH SURVEILLANCE

When a community in the United States has a question about how their environment might be impacting their health, public health practitioners often don't have much data to draw upon to answer it.

Megan Latshaw, Assistant Scientist

Johns Hopkins Bloomberg School of Public Health

Dr. Latshaw focuses on designing healthy communities, connecting environmental health research and the real world, and improving environmental health data collection. At Johns Hopkins, Dr. Latshaw teaches and directs two master's degree programs. She serves as co-lead of the Environmental Challenges Focus Area of the Bloomberg American Health Initiative, and she is a past chair of the American Public Health Association's Environment Section.

What do you see as the greatest issues regarding environmental health surveillance in urban areas, what are the major obstacles to addressing these issues, and what is your hope for the future?

Everything around us impacts our health—from the air we breathe to the water we use, the food we eat, and the neighborhoods in which we live. However, environmental health lacks a comprehensive national state-based system for collecting and analyzing data. Thus, when a community in the United States has a question about how their environment might be impacting their health, public health practitioners often don't have much data to draw upon to answer it. This is especially true in comparison to our country's relatively strong infectious and chronic disease surveillance systems.

For environmental health, the Centers for Disease Control and Prevention's (CDC's) Environmental Public Health Tracking Network represents a national surveillance system. It collects, integrates, analyzes, interprets, and disseminates information from environmental hazard monitoring, human exposure, and health effects data. But this tracking network only includes 26 health departments (mostly state-based), and analysis at the local level remains limited. On the human exposure side, the National Health and Nutrition Examination Survey provides some data on the concentration of chemicals in Americans' blood and urine, but these data cannot be resolved at the state or local levels. The CDC's state-based Biomonitoring Program aims to build this ability at the state and local levels, but it currently only covers nine states.

The National Biomonitoring Network aims to build a state-based environmental health surveillance system that can be used to address community environmental health questions. It builds upon the Tracking Network, the Biomonitoring Program, and the CDC's Laboratory Response Network, where investments in preparedness have created advanced chemistry capabilities in 45 state and local laboratories across the country.

A comprehensive environmental health surveillance system can not only help to answer community questions about the impact of the environment on their health, but it can also increase our understanding of chemical exposures at the state and local levels, improve our ability to measure the impact of public health interventions or environmental policies, and increase the efficient use of resources for cleaning up environmental contamination.

Climate Change

The earth's climate is always changing—it has been ever since the atmosphere first formed. What is different now is that the change is happening rapidly, so much so that scientists are uncertain whether the earth's natural systems and life forms, which evolved slowly over time, can adapt to the abruptly rising temperatures and other climate aberrations expected before the end of this century. According to the World Health Organization (WHO), climate change is already causing tens of thousands of deaths every year, mainly from shifting patterns of disease, extreme weather events, and degradation of air quality, food, water supplies, and sanitation. People living in cities are particularly vulnerable to the effects of climate change, such as heat waves and air pollution, flooding of coastal communities, and the spread of infectious diseases. Around the globe, average temperatures are rising almost everywhere.

Scientists have used several approaches to estimate what the earth's climate was like as far back as a million years ago. By analyzing ice cores, tree rings, glacier lengths, pollen remains, ocean sediments, and changes in the earth's orbit, researchers have documented how the earth's climate has varied due to natural causes, such as (1) changes in solar energy; (2) variations in naturally occurring greenhouse gas (GHG) concentrations in the atmosphere; and (3) periodic volcanic eruptions that eject large quantities of particles and gases into the air. However, the climatic changes that have occurred since the Industrial Revolution cannot be explained by natural causes alone. Instead, changes this significant could only have happened due to human activities.

The principal human activities leading to climate change involve the combustion of fossil fuels—coal, oil, and natural gas—to generate electricity, power our motor vehicles, and provide energy for industrial operations. These activities, which tend to concentrate in urban areas, emit large quantities of air pollutants, particularly the principal GHG, carbon dioxide (CO_2), into the atmosphere. Other industrial and commercial activities, including oil and gas, landfill, livestock, and agricultural operations, also produce significant amounts of GHGs. Deforestation—the large-scale clearing of forests taking place in some parts of the world—contributes to climate change because forests are natural carbon sinks. Additionally, warming of the atmosphere can occur when the earth's surface is modified (e.g., when natural areas are paved with heat-absorbing asphalt and concrete as urban areas expand). Some natural phenomena, such as volcanic eruptions and forest fires, also contribute to climate change, but human activities remain the dominant cause, particularly during the twentieth century and up to the present time.

While most global warming associated with human activities is caused by CO_2, other air pollutants contributing to climate change include methane, nitrous oxide, and some fluorinated gases, such as hydrofluorocarbons, perfluorocarbons, sulfur hexafluoride, and nitrogen trifluoride. Working together, these gases act like a blanket, holding warm temperatures close to the earth's surface and preventing heat from escaping to outer space. This is called the "greenhouse effect" because the GHGs trap heat close to the earth's surface, similar to how a greenhouse allows sunlight to pass through its transparent ceiling and walls but prevents much of the heat inside from escaping.

Solutions to climate change are not so simple because even if all the nations of the world agreed to cease their CO_2 emissions immediately, some CO_2 already emitted into the atmosphere would remain there for thousands of years, due in part to the slow process by which atmospheric carbon is transferred to the oceans and ocean sediments. While several techniques have been proposed to remove CO_2 from the atmosphere and to reuse it or store it underground, most scientists are skeptical about the efficacy of these techniques over a reasonable time frame. Thus, climate change occurring this century may require centuries more time to reverse. This explains the urgency felt by many nations to address climate change now. Figure 1, which illustrates the year-to-year increase in CO_2 concentrations in the atmosphere observed since 1958, demonstrates that current global policies to reduce CO_2 concentrations are not working.

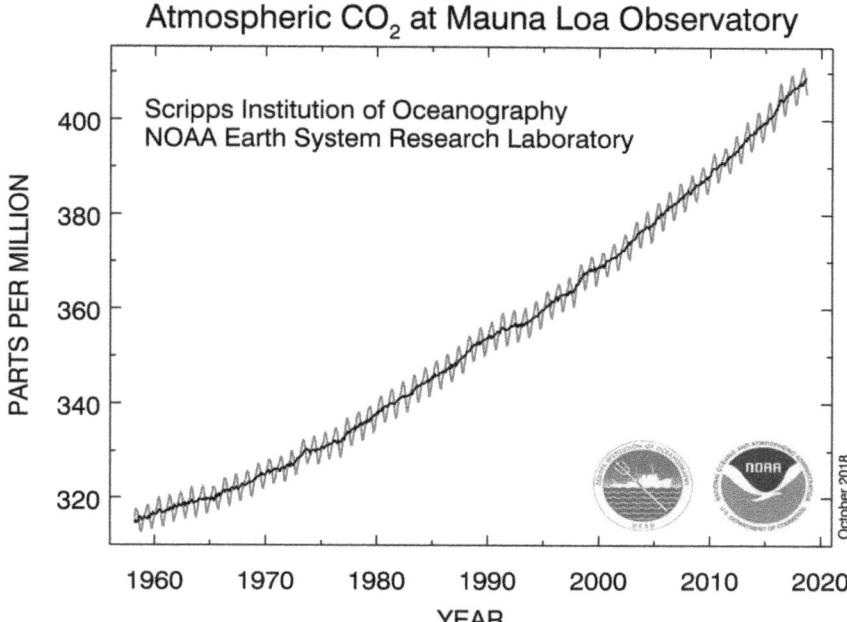

Figure 1   Monthly mean atmospheric CO_2 concentrations at the Mauna Loa Observatory, 1958–2018. The dark curve represents seasonally corrected data. (*Source*: National Oceanic and Atmospheric Administration.)

Most climate scientists believe that cities are already experiencing climate change effects, including longer heat waves, more flooding, and degraded air quality from nearby forest fires, and there is concern that warmer temperatures will cause the territories of mosquitoes and other disease-carrying vectors to expand, spreading diseases to highly populated urban areas. In the United States, record-breaking temperatures are becoming more commonplace, and several regions have suffered unprecedented flooding. For example, the subway system in New York City was paralyzed in 2016 when flooding occurred from intense rainfall, stranding 2.5 million riders, and in 2017, the streets of Houston were inundated for weeks when Hurricane Harvey dumped over 50 inches (127 centimeters) of rain, causing 68 deaths. In 2018, severe flooding in Japan, unlike anything ever seen before, resulted in nearly 200 deaths, and the rapid intensification of Hurricane Michael, one of the strongest hurricanes ever to strike the United States, was attributed to unusually warm Gulf of Mexico waters related to climate change. Meanwhile, some cities like Cape Town, South Africa, are running out of drinking water due to climate change–related drought. Mathematical climate models predict that global warming will continue, with no end in sight, unless the nations of the world act expeditiously to reduce GHG emissions.

IMPACT ON URBAN HEALTH

The ways in which climate change will affect the health of city dwellers are not fully understood, but public health experts have been studying this issue very carefully and have developed several dire scenarios for human health and the spread of disease later this century. In the United States, the American Public Health Association is deeply concerned about climate change health effects, declaring 2017 the Year of Climate Change and Health. And the WHO reports that although climate change may have some localized benefits, such as fewer wintertime deaths in temperate climates and increased food production in some regions, "the overall health effects of a changing climate are likely to be overwhelmingly negative."

Some of the predicted effects of climate change and consequences for human health, particularly in urban environments, include the following:

- **Droughts, heavy rainfall, and flooding events**—As these events increase in frequency, intensity, and duration, livelihoods will be disrupted (particularly jobs in agriculture) and waterborne diseases will spread. People living in submarginal housing will suffer from greater exposure to the elements, and fresh water may be in short supply for many regions of the world. Agricultural production may decline, causing widespread malnutrition and famine in villages and larger urban areas and potentially resulting in the displacement of large populations.

- **Extreme heat events**—More illness and death will result from higher temperatures, especially in urban areas, which tend to be hotter than surrounding rural areas. Hospital emergency room admissions will increase on unusually hot days, and older adults will be particularly at risk from the stifling city heat. When combined with city air pollution, higher temperatures will cause more cardiovascular disease and stroke.

- **Infectious diseases**—By lengthening the transmission seasons and altering the range of mosquitoes and other disease vectors, climate change will cause infectious diseases to increase and spread rapidly to populated urban areas.

- **Ozone air pollution**—The ozone pollution found in many metropolitan areas will worsen due to the warmer temperatures caused by climate change, resulting in increased respiratory symptoms and aggravated lung diseases (e.g., asthma, emphysema, and chronic bronchitis) and making the lungs more susceptible to infection. Chronic exposure to higher levels of ozone will magnify certain serious health problems, such as chronic obstructive pulmonary disease (COPD).
- **Pollen and other aeroallergens**—As the climate warms, asthma and other respiratory ailments associated with aeroallergens will likely increase, and the heat and pollution present in urban areas will tend to aggravate these illnesses.
- **Rising sea levels**—Homes and businesses in low-lying areas that are inundated by seawater will be abandoned, resulting in economic losses, and local communities will be disrupted. Increases in depression and other mental disorders would be expected.

Many unknowns remain about how climate change will affect health in urban environments. For example, how severely will climate change affect the most vulnerable individuals—children, older adults, pregnant women, communities of color, indigenous communities, outdoor workers, and people with disabilities and chronic medical conditions? As climate change becomes more severe, will chronic mental stress develop among tens of millions of city residents around the world, causing increased susceptibility to disease? Will weather extremes result in increased pesticide use, causing more human exposure to toxic chemicals on fruits and vegetables? The answers to these questions will depend in part on how severe the climate change crisis becomes and whether the nations of the world can come together to implement rigorous global GHG-reduction policies and programs.

WHAT CITIES ARE DOING ABOUT CLIMATE CHANGE

Although cities cover just 2 percent of the earth's surface, they are responsible for over 60 percent of CO_2 emissions. Cities are particularly vulnerable to climate change due to their large and growing populations and extensive infrastructure systems. These systems are often a complex array of interconnected services—water and wastewater treatment facilities, energy plants, transportation systems, and data management and telecommunications centers—that in many cases are aging and in urgent need of repair. Recognizing these vulnerabilities, cities have been particularly pro-active in the fight against climate change, sometimes more so than their national governments. Some cities have also found that urban planning and development, based on green, environmentally friendly principles that reduce GHGs, create a more pleasant cityscape that is good for tourism and commercial investment.

To address climate change, many city governments are striving to reduce the "heat island effect," a term that describes how urban areas are often hotter than their surroundings due to the ability of dense building and paving materials, like concrete, asphalt, brick, stone, and steel, to absorb and retain heat from the sun. As temperatures rise due to climate change, the heat island effect will only worsen, contributing to longer and more severe heat waves and more heat-related health illness and mortality. Cities are countering the heat island effect by planting native, drought-tolerant shade trees, installing green (vegetation-covered) roofs on city buildings, and shading building surfaces from the hot summer sun. Additionally, many cities are developing or expanding public parks and greenways to provide cooler surfaces, shading, and a natural means of filtering air pollution and stormwater runoff. These greenways often serve as pedestrian corridors, where people can walk or ride bicycles to work, school, or shopping areas without having to depend on personal vehicles and public transportation.

Many cities are improving their urban transportation infrastructure, such as providing more low-polluting bus and commuter rail routes and encouraging compact building practices (i.e., placing buildings closer together), particularly for urban infill projects. By improving public trans-portation options and locating housing, jobs, schools, shopping, and parks in close proximity, city residents are less dependent on their personal vehi-cles, with the result that GHGs and other urban pollutants are reduced. To further address climate change concerns, many cities incorporate energy efficiency into their building codes (e.g., specifying performance require-ments for heating and air conditioning, building insulation, and windows), and some cities encourage renewable energy technologies, such as photo-voltaic (solar) cells and solar hot water heaters. An increasing number of new buildings are designed to achieve Leadership in Energy and Environ-mental Design standards and other green building certifications.

As 100-year floods are occurring with increasing frequency, several times per decade in some cases, cities are becoming increasing aware that their old flood maps need to be redrawn and zoning laws updated to prevent new building construction in flood-prone areas. Furthermore, many coastal communities are experiencing regular high-tide and storm-surge flooding to an extent not previously seen. These flooding events will increase in severity in the coming years as climate change raises sea levels and modifies weather patterns, causing a greater number of heavy rainfall events from storms, hurricanes, and typhoons. To address these concerns, many cities have been upgrading their water supply and stormwater draining systems, relocating energy and waste management facilities to higher ground, building seawalls to block rising ocean waters, and replacing concrete and asphalt surfaces with grass and other permeable surfaces to absorb water runoff.

RECOMMENDATIONS FOR CITY DWELLERS

For protection against the effects of climate change, urban dwellers should avoid going outside on hot days, and when they do go out, they should stay in the shade as much as possible, wear long-sleeve shirts and long pants, and use sunscreen lotion. Also, people should avoid outdoor activities when the air quality is poor. In addition, it is important to try to stay healthy during the flu season, when infectious diseases can spread more easily, by practicing good hygiene (e.g., handwashing), getting a flu shot, avoiding large crowds, and staying away from people showing symptoms of an infection. For city residents with asthma or allergies that worsen during heat waves and air pollution episodes, they should monitor outdoor conditions (e.g., daily pollen counts) and consult with their doctor about precautions to remain healthy.

One of the most important steps that urban residents can take to fight climate change is to educate their elected representatives about the threat to public health and severe economic consequences from a warming climate, especially for cities that will have to bear the burden of remedial response at the local level. When communicating with elected officials, residents should stress the importance of mobilizing the world's nations to set common goals to reduce GHGs, aided by international treaties and accords. On a more local scale, there are actions that individuals can take at home and in their neighborhoods to fight climate change, as noted in Table 3.

Table 3   Actions to Fight Climate Change at Home and in Your Community

Location	Actions to Fight Climate Change
At home	• To save energy, buy energy-efficient lighting and appliances (e.g., those carrying the *Energy Star* label).
	• Reduce heating and cooling costs by changing air filters regularly, using a programmable thermostat, and performing routine maintenance on the furnace and air conditioner.
	• Prevent energy from leaking to the outside of the house by applying caulking and weather stripping around doors and windows and installing insulation in walls, ceilings, and floors, as needed.
	• Practice the three Rs—reduce, reuse, and recycle—to cut down on waste and GHG emissions from resource extraction, manufacturing, and landfill operations. Composting food and yard waste helps too.
	• Reduce domestic water use, which can help to reduce GHG emissions by cutting back on the energy needed to pump and treat water at municipal treatment works. For example, fix leaky toilets, do not run water while brushing teeth, only operate the dishwasher and washing machine with full loads, and limit unnecessary lawn and landscape watering.
	• Where available, buy green power, which is electricity generated from renewable energy sources, including solar cells and wind turbines.
At work	• Reduce energy consumption by turning off computers, printers, copiers, and other office equipment when not in use. (Some equipment can be set to turn off or go into sleep mode at night or after a period of inactivity.) Be sure to purchase only certified energy-efficient office equipment.
	• Travel to and from work using public transportation, a carpool, or a bicycle, or walk to work if you live close enough. (Some employers provide transportation incentives, such as subsidies for riding the bus or other public transportation or special parking spaces for carpools.) If you must drive, purchase a fuel-efficient car.

Table 3   (continued)

Location	Actions to Fight Climate Change
	• Reduce waste at work by printing and copying only when necessary, doing two-sided printing and copying, and recycling paper and printer ink cartridges.
	• When upgrading equipment, reduce landfill waste by recycling it or donating the equipment to organizations such as schools and nonprofits.
	• Work with your managers to develop an office GHG inventory, which can help identify activities and equipment that needlessly consume energy. (Some companies are surprised to discover that simple steps to reduce energy use also can reduce company operating costs.)
While driving	• Purchase a low-emission, fuel-efficient, or electric vehicle, and try to limit driving by walking, bicycling, or taking public transportation.
	• Reduce gasoline use by accelerating and braking slowly, reducing idling time, and using cruise control on freeways.
	• Perform regular maintenance to keep your engine operating optimally.
	• Check to be sure that your tires are not underinflated because when the tire pressure is low, fuel economy can suffer. When buying new tires, consider ones have low rolling resistance, a feature that can improve fuel economy.
	• Use renewable fuel blends, such as E85 (85 percent ethanol and 15 percent gasoline) or biodiesel blends, provided that your car or truck is designed to run on these fuels.

CITY SPOTLIGHT: VENICE—WILL ANYTHING WORK TO STOP THE FLOODING?

Flooding has become more common in the streets of Venice, as climate change raises sea levels and water infiltrates the city at high tide. Tourism and public health and safety depend on finding a workable solution.

Venice is one of the world's most popular vacation spots, with 25 million tourists visiting this Italian city every year to experience the ubiquitous canals, picturesque bridges, and renowned works of art. But Venice faces two serious problems that threaten the city's architectural treasures and the health and safety of its citizens: It is sinking, and climate change is making that situation worse. Natural land subsistence combined with rising water levels caused by global warming have combined to make Venice more vulnerable to flooding than any time in its past.

Many older Venetians remember the horrific flooding of November 1966, when strong offshore winds and heavy rains combined with high tidal waves to cause severe flooding, lasting two days and reaching heights of 76 inches (194 centimeters) above sea level. At times, the floodwater covered the entire city, doing great damage to the historic center, ruining precious works of art, and forcing residents to seek refuge on higher floors and rooftops. When it was over, streets were littered with dead rats, electricity service was out, food spoiled, and residents faced a desperate situation. More than a dozen people died, and thousands were left homeless. The floodwater also invaded nearby towns and villages, ultimately claiming the lives of over 100 people in the region.

To prevent a recurrence of the historic 1966 flooding, engineers began studying in earnest potential solutions, but the complexity of the problem was overwhelming. Estimates vary, but the city is believed to have sunk between 5 and 10 inches (13–25 centimeters) during the last century, partly caused by the construction of wells near the lagoon that surrounds Venice, removing vast quantities of groundwater needed by local factories. The wells were eventually banned, and the rate of subsistence declined. However, the city is still slowly sinking, and there is little that can be done about it. At the same time, the neighboring Adriatic Sea continues rising from climate change, and high-tide flooding of the city is becoming more frequent.

City officials eventually settled on an approach to solving the flooding problem, which is to build a series of 78 retractable floodgates across the three inlets to Venice's lagoon. The idea is simple: Hollow floodgates lie on the seabed, weighed down by water inside the gates. When city flooding is imminent, the water is pumped out of the gates and replaced with air, allowing the now-buoyant floodgates to rise to the surface, where they block the incoming tide. After the flood threat has passed, the gates are again filled with water, and they sink back down to the bottom of the sea. The cycle repeats every time the city is threatened with flooding.

The floodgate project, known as Modulo Sperimentale Elettromeccanico ("MOSE" for short), has been plagued by cost overruns and design issues, and several dozen people connected to the project, including the mayor of Venice, were arrested for bribery and bid-rigging, among other charges. As a result, the floodgate project has been delayed time and again. Begun in 2003, the project is headed toward completion in the 2019–2020 time frame. But with its history of delays, the actual startup date remains uncertain.

Also uncertain is how long MOSE will actually protect the city. The project was designed for a 50-year lifespan, but with the current rate of sea level rise and tidal flooding, the useful life of MOSE may be closer to three decades. Much depends on the severity of climate change and the political will of nations to cut back on GHG emissions through global agreements like the 2015 Paris climate agreement. Current climate change calculations indicate that even without the tides, the entire city of Venice may be continuously underwater within a century if global warming continues with little abatement.

In addition to the floodgates, other measures are being taken to defend the city against flooding. These include dredging the canals to allow better water exchange in the inner lagoon, managing runoff from industrial areas, reinforcing existing seawalls, and restoring the salt marshes. Many cities around the world are paying close attention to Venice's flood-management experiment to see what lessons can be applied to their own situations. There is concern in the United States that over 650 coastal communities may experience chronic flooding from climate change by the end of the century, potentially displacing countless residences and businesses, and in Europe, about 86 million people living within 6 miles (10 kilometers) of a coastline are at risk of coastal flooding. There are similar worries throughout the rest of the world, including predictions that parts of Fiji, Tonga, the Cook Islands, and other South Pacific island nations may soon be submerged below rising ocean waters. Several small islands that are part of the archipelago that constitutes the Solomon Islands have already disappeared due to rising seas and erosion.

Crime and Violence

Crime and violence are unfortunate facts of city life. In many large metropolitan areas, hardly a day passes without news reports about criminal activity and gang violence, often related to drugs and alcohol. However, although large cities can be breeding grounds for crime and violence, smaller towns are not immune, and even rural areas can have per capita crime and violence rates comparable to bigger cities. Thus, the common belief that cities are so much more dangerous than rural areas is a myth in many parts of the world. Nevertheless, cities experience large numbers of crimes because of their size, and they often have pockets of crime-ridden areas to be avoided.

According to the World Health Organization (WHO), 1.4 million deaths occur every year due to violence (including almost a half-million homicides), and for every person who dies, there are countless other cases of injury and suffering from a range of physical, sexual, and mental health abuse. Often, this violence is associated with criminal activity, but it can also result from domestic and workplace violence, child and elder abuse, violence against women, and the effects of drugs and alcohol. The economic toll of violence on the world's economy resulting from increased healthcare and law enforcement costs and lost worker productivity is measured in billions of U.S. dollars.

Globally, over 80 percent of violence-related deaths are caused by homicide and suicide, problems that have plagued large cities for years. About half of these deaths are suicides, one-third result from violent injuries caused by another person, and around 10 percent are associated with war or some other collective conflict. (The WHO includes suicide in its statistics on violence, considering it a form of violence against oneself.) Countries having high levels of economic inequality tend to have more deaths due to violence, and death rates are often highest in the poorest communities. Most deaths due to violence occur among young men aged 15–44 in low- and middle-income countries, and for every such death, an estimated 20–40 young people incur injuries requiring hospitalization. For every suicide death among people under 25 years old, there are 100 attempted suicides.

In the United States, variations in the number of violent crimes and less serious property offenses occur from year to year, but generally, these rates have been declining since peaking in the early 1990s. (While murder and violent crimes rates rose slightly in 2015 and 2016, these rates are falling again, and there is no evidence that the country is experiencing a crime wave, as some fear.) There are various theories for the declining U.S. crime rate, including increased policing, but many experts believe that economic factors, such as job creation and urban redevelopment, play an important role.

According to the U.S. Federal Bureau of Investigation (FBI), there were about 1.2 million violent crimes (i.e., murder and nonnegligent manslaughter, rape, robbery, and aggravated assault) in 2017, or close to 400 violent criminal offenses for every 100,000 residents. Over the same period, there were about 7.7 million property crimes (i.e., burglary, larceny-theft, and motor vehicle theft), with an economic impact of over $15 billion. However, crime and violence estimates are probably underestimated because less than half of violent crimes and only one-third of property crimes are reported to police, according to the Bureau of Justice Statistics. Table 4 summarizes the types of violent and property crimes in the United States as a percent of total crimes.

A 2016 study by Grinshteyn and Hemenway in the *American Journal of Medicine* found that U.S. homicide rates were 7 times higher than in other high-income countries, and homicides by firearms were 25 times higher. Homicide is a serious issue in the United States, and a great debate is raging about the role of firearms. For example, proponents of more stringent gun control laws argue that such laws would reduce gun deaths, whereas opponents argue that gun ownership helps deter crime. The debate also centers around interpretations of the Second Amendment to the U.S. Constitution (concerning the right to bear arms) and the degree to which it protects individual gun ownership. The Pew Research Center reported in 2017 that 30 percent of U.S. adults own a gun; 44 percent say that they

Table 4   Violent and Property Crimes in the United States

Crime	Percent of Total
Violent Crimes	
Aggravated assault	65
Robbery	26
Rape	8
Murder	1
Property Crimes	
Larceny-theft (excluding motor vehicles)	72
Burglary	18
Motor vehicle theft	10

Source: Federal Bureau of Investigation (FBI), 2017. (Arson data are excluded because of reporting variations among agencies.)

personally know someone who has been shot, either accidentally or intentionally; and 15 percent say that they have fired or threatened to fire a gun to defend themselves, their family members, or their possessions. While there are sharp divides among those who own guns and those who do not, a strong majority of both groups favor limiting access to guns for people with mental illnesses and individuals who are on the federal terrorist watch and no-fly lists.

Crime and violence can affect anyone living in the city, but there are special concerns for several groups of citizens who are more vulnerable and at greater risk, as follows:

• **Violence against children**—As many as 1 billion children age 2–17 experience physical, sexual, or emotional violence or neglect per year, according to the WHO. Violence can be perpetrated by parents, other caregivers, peers, romantic partners, or strangers; and forms of violence include maltreatment (e.g., violent punishment, neglect, negligence, and commercial exploitation), bullying (including cyberbullying), youth and gang violence, intimate partner and other domestic violence, and sexual violence (e.g., sexual harassment, sexual trafficking, and online exploitation). About 25 percent of adults report having been physically abused as children, including one in five women reporting sexual abuse.

- **Youth violence**—Over 40 percent of global homicides occur among young adults age 10–29, representing the fourth-leading cause of death in this age group. Over 80 percent of these victims are males. Assaults often involve physical fighting and bullying with fists, feet, knives, and blunt objects, and it is no surprise that assaults involving firearms cause the greatest number of fatal injuries. For every death from violence, there may be thousands of incidents resulting in hospitalization and potentially serious psychological effects that last a lifetime.

- **Violence against women**—Violence against women includes acts of gender-based violence causing or likely to cause physical, sexual, or mental harm or suffering. The WHO reports that about one-third of all women worldwide who have been in an intimate relationship have experienced physical or sexual violence by their partner, and up to 38 percent of murders of women are committed by a male intimate partner. Women are also frequently subjected to violence by others, including relatives, acquaintances, and strangers.

- **Elder abuse**—When an older adult is subjected to physical, sexual, psychological, or emotional abuse, or when material and financial needs have been neglected or restricted, elder abuse has occurred. Such abuse often happens where there is an expectation of trust with a caregiver, and often the older adult suffers a loss of dignity and respect. According to the WHO, around 15 percent of adults age 60 and older experienced some form of abuse in home and other community settings, and the abuse may be even greater in institutional settings, such as hospitals, nursing homes, and long-term-care facilities. Cases of elder abuse may be underestimated because older adults are hesitant to report abuse to family, friends, or the authorities. Elder abuse will become a more serious global issue in the future, as the number of people age 60 and older is expected to double by 2050.

- **Violence against healthcare workers**—Nurses and other staff members involved with patient care, including emergency room workers and paramedics, are at a particularly high risk of violence. Between 8 and 38 percent of healthcare workers are believed to have experienced physical violence at some point during their careers, the WHO reports, and many more have been subjected to verbal aggression. This violence is mainly perpetrated by patients and visitors, but healthcare workers are also injured while providing care during civil unrest, political violence, and conflicts between nations.

- **Suicide**—Nearly 800,000 people worldwide take their lives every year, and many more attempt suicide. While suicide happens everywhere, about 80 percent of the cases occur in low- and middle-income countries, where the most common methods are ingestion of pesticides, hanging, and use of a firearm. In the United States, the most common methods of suicide are use of a firearm, suffocation, and poisoning. Suicide is particularly a problem for U.S. military veterans, who take their own lives at the rate that may approach 18 to 22 per day by some estimates. Veterans account for around 7 percent of the U.S. adult population, but 18 percent of all suicide deaths.

IMPACT ON URBAN HEALTH

In addition to physical injury and death, crime and violence can have both physical and emotional long-term effects. For example, victims of serious crimes and physical violence have increased rates of depression and other mental disorders, suicide, chronic pain, unwanted pregnancies, and sexually transmitted infections. And these effects may lead to work productivity and communication problems, loss of a job, and considerable stress on family life.

Crime and violence can be particularly hard on children. At an early age, exposure to violence can impair brain development, leading to poor cognitive development and underachievement in school, and it can damage the nervous, endocrine, circulatory, musculoskeletal, reproductive, respiratory, and immune systems. Furthermore, the negative coping and health-risk behaviors resulting from violence can lead to an increased risk for cardiovascular disease, cancer, diabetes, and other health problems as the child grows older. (The term "toxic stress" is often applied to stressful situations, such as physical or emotional abuse and neglect and exposure to violence, that activate stress-response systems in children and can increase the risk for disease and cognitive impairment, sometimes lasting well into adulthood.) Children exposed to violence are more likely to smoke, abuse drugs and alcohol, engage in high-risk sexual behavior, drop out of school, attempt suicide, and suffer from obesity, anxiety, and depression; and these children are also at an increased risk of victimization and interpersonal violence later in life. Table 5 illustrates the dose-response relationship between adverse childhood experiences (e.g., violence, abuse, and neglect) and health and well-being outcomes later in life, and Table 6 lists seven global strategies for ending violence against children.

Table 5   Dose-Response Relationship Between Adverse Childhood Experiences and Health and Well-Being Outcomes

As the Number of Adverse Childhood Experiences Increases, So Does the Risk Later in Life for the Following:[a]

- Adolescent pregnancy
- Alcoholism and alcohol abuse
- Chronic obstructive pulmonary disease (COPD)
- Depression
- Early initiation of sexual activity
- Early initiation of smoking
- Fetal death
- Financial stress
- Health-related quality of life
- Illicit drug use
- Ischemic heart disease
- Liver disease
- Multiple sexual partners
- Poor academic achievement
- Poor work performance
- Risk of intimate partner violence
- Risk of sexual violence
- Sexually transmitted diseases
- Smoking
- Suicide attempts
- Unintended pregnancies

[a]Adverse childhood experiences are incidents involving violence, abuse, and neglect.

Source: Centers for Disease Control and Prevention (CDC) and Kaiser Permanente, Adverse Childhood Experiences Study.

Even without crime and violence, life in the city can be challenging for many residents who are forced to work two or more jobs to make ends meet, all while raising children and possibly caring for older parents as well. When a violent crime affects a family member, in addition to the physical and mental harm caused, the family member may lose employment, undergo expensive medical treatments, or suffer from depression. This can be hard on everyone in the family, resulting in anxiety-related illnesses, discord among family members, and possible abuse of drugs and alcohol.

WHAT CITIES ARE DOING ABOUT CRIME AND VIOLENCE

While crime remains a serious problem in many urban areas, some cities have witnessed a remarkable decline in crime in recent years. The reasons for this are not altogether clear, although economic growth, urban

Table 6   Global Strategies for Ending Violence against Children

Strategy	Examples
Implementing and enforcing laws	Banning violent discipline and restricting access to alcohol and firearms
Changing norms and values	Altering norms that condone the sexual abuse of girls or aggressive behavior among boys
Fostering safe environments	Identifying neighborhood hot spots for violence, and then addressing the local causes through problem-oriented policing and other interventions
Encouraging parental and caregiver support	Providing parent training to young, first-time parents
Increasing income and economic strengthening	Offering microfinancing and gender-equity training
Providing response services	Ensuring that children who are exposed to violence can access effective emergency care and receive appropriate psychosocial support
Offering education and training in life skills	Ensuring that children attend school and providing life and social skills training

Source: WHO.

redevelopment and revitalization, and low unemployment in many areas are undoubtedly important factors. Realizing that brute force is no longer a very effective deterrent, police departments have gotten much smarter in how they approach crime prevention and mobilize local community support, even as they increase their focus on gun violence and shutting down drug markets. Communities have learned to take more ownership over their local crime problems, working with nonprofit organizations to provide drug counseling, youth mentoring, community education, and job creation. Funding for intervention and education from foundations and the private sector also has proved to be very effective in helping communities address local crime and violence problems. Another factor in the reduced crime rate is the proliferation of home and automobile security systems and private security guards at commercial operations.

There may be lessons to be learned from large American cities like Chicago, which has been struggling with rampant gang violence that at times has seemed uncontrollable. Gun violence in Chicago is particularly a problem, with homicides reported daily and several thousand nonfatal gun-related injuries occurring every year. The violence is worse in communities experiencing high rates of poverty and joblessness, suggesting that local economics may be an important factor. Building on successful crime-prevention programs in other cities, such as New York City and Los Angeles, Chicago has implemented a multifaceted crime-reduction program aimed at reducing gang violence and returning a sense of safety to the city's neighborhoods, and since implementing this program, the city has witnessed a significant reduction in gun violence. (Homicides were down 15 percent from 2016 to 2017.) Chicago's approach to crime and violence reduction includes the following:

- Hiring more police officers, empowering district commanders to respond quickly to criminal behavior based on their analysis of local crime patterns, and implementing hot-spot policing, which involves daily analyses of areas or situations likely to experience violence

- Using technology and data analytics as crime-fighting tools, and installing a high-tech strategic-decision support center to help target crime

- Closely monitoring gang rivalries, and targeting criminals with guns as a major focus of law enforcement

- Outfitting officers with body-worn video cameras, providing more Tasers to reduce the number of deadly confrontations, and improving officer training in conflict resolution, de-escalation, and use of force

- Creating a citizens' oversight board to monitor police department activities and recommend improvements, working with community and church groups to involve former gang members in resolving conflicts, and collaborating with community organizers to provide mentoring for children living in the most troubled areas

- Improving economic opportunities by encouraging commercial businesses to invest in marginal and distressed neighborhoods, and launching a neighborhood-opportunity fund that permits higher-density developments near downtown areas in return for funds for further economic development and job training.

As with other cities that have successfully fought crime, Chicago's approach includes a mixture of better policing and police oversight, urban development, job creation, and mentoring for at-risk youth, and improving police morale is also considered a key to success. Some of these approaches will undoubtedly bear fruit, while others may not, but through aggressive program implementation and experimentation, and by continued monitoring of crime-reduction successes in other cities, Chicago is learning how to manage its crime problem, perhaps one day becoming a model for other cities.

RECOMMENDATIONS FOR CITY DWELLERS

To help reduce crime and violence in their neighborhoods, urban dwellers can get involved with community organizations that fight crime (e.g., through educational or mentoring programs). Mentoring a youngster or becoming a big brother or sister can help prevent criminal behavior and have a lasting impact on a child's development and success as an adult. Other actions to help reduce neighborhood crime and violence include attending public hearings on crime, voting for candidates who are concerned about preventing crime and seem to be effective at it, and talking with local police about crime and violence prevention. By supporting an organization like Neighborhood Watch (a crime-prevention program where citizens learn how to identify and report suspicious activity in their neighborhoods), people can join with their neighbors in watching for criminal behavior and reporting it to the police.

Here are some common-sense actions that urban dwellers can take to protect themselves from crime and violence:

- Walk with a purpose, look like you know where you are going, do not ask people on the street for directions, and avoid talking on your cell phone because it signals criminals that you are distracted and may not see them approach you.
- If you are going out at night, particularly alone, let a friend or family member know where you are going and for how long, so that they can notify the police if you do not return on time.
- In entertainment districts, go with friends (not alone), avoid wearing expensive clothing and jewelry, and park your car in a well-lit lot or garage with an attendant.
- Be careful about drinking in public because your judgment can be affected and predators may misinterpret your intentions toward them.
- Carry valuables in an inside pocket, and be careful about purses with shoulder straps that can fling you to the ground if a criminal grabs the purse.

- When using an automated teller machine (ATM), make sure that no one is watching you or hovering nearby, and do not count your money in public areas.

- Sit near the front of a bus, never enter an empty subway car, and if driving, get in your car quickly, checking that no one is hiding in the back seat.

- Consider taking a self-defense course, carrying a defensive product like pepper spray or a personal alarm, and getting a dog with a loud bark.

- Keep your home front door locked, beware of phone scams, and never give out personal or financial information over the phone.

- Always be aware of your surroundings and trust your instincts to avoid an area or situation that does not feel right.

Remember to take charge of your own safety by staying alert, watching your surroundings, and being careful about subtle, nonverbal cues that can make you appear vulnerable, like looking nervous or lost or having a downward gaze. By taking reasonable precautions and being smart about preventing crime, people living in the city can avoid most threatening situations and reduce the risk of being targeted.

CITY SPOTLIGHT: NEW YORK CITY—AN INTERNATIONAL MODEL OF CRIMINAL JUSTICE REFORM

America's largest city has experienced a dramatic reduction in crime. The reasons are complex and multifaceted, but changing attitudes about crime and the role of community organizations appear to be critical to this success.

The crime rate in New York City is way down, and so is the jail population. By 2018, the number of people incarcerated in the city had slipped below 9,000—down from 20,000 in the mid-1980s. There are many theories for the city's declining crime rate—economic growth and urban revitalization, a reduction in crack cocaine use, demographic changes, lower childhood lead exposure, and improvements in policing practices. However, experts caution that the story is not so simple, and a variety of policies and strategies have come together over time to cut crime to the levels experienced today.

One important factor is believed to be the proliferation of community crime prevention initiatives, like the Cure Violence model, which treats violence more like a disease epidemic. This approach to fighting crime involves strategies aimed at detecting and interrupting conflicts, identifying and treating the highest-risk individuals, and changing social norms. For example, the program addresses negative peer pressure, instills in young people the courage to walk away from a fight, and creates expectations of peaceful conflict resolution within the community. Community organizations are also working to educate the public and mediate conflict, sometimes by mobilizing people who were once caught up in criminal behavior themselves, but now want to help others avoid criminal acts and improve community life. This type of community outreach and local activism tackles the crime problem while avoiding excessive policing and helping reduce the incarceration rate.

Another successful approach to fighting crime and violence in New York City is to provide alternatives to incarceration that help build the self-esteem of offenders and give them a second chance at living a normal, law-abiding life. Using this strategy, the city has created a number of special courts that sentence defendants to drug-treatment programs rather than jail, and there is solid evidence that these courts have been successful in reducing drug abuse and preventing backsliding toward repeat criminal behavior. Other programs replace jail sentences and fines with social and community service and direct mentally ill defendants to get counseling. Such programs are based on the theory that jail time does little to address the underlying causes of crime, and by giving criminal offenders an opportunity and framework for re-creating their lives, many end their criminal activities and learn to contribute to their communities in positive ways.

The city has also been successful in implementing the concept of procedural justice (also called "procedural fairness"), which is the idea that offenders are more likely to comply with police or court orders and avoid future criminal behavior if they respect the judicial process, perceive that their treatment is fair, and feel that they were treated with dignity and respect. Even if the criminal offender disagrees with the ultimate judicial ruling, the rate of compliance with court orders goes up, and future criminal behavior goes down. The key concepts of procedural justice include (1) humanizing the experience; (2) explaining in clear language the judicial process and why it is happening; (3) providing opportunities for the accused to express their views and be heard in the judicial process; and (4) improving environmental factors, such as creating more pleasant and less dehumanizing criminal justice facilities, with features such as signs in multiple languages. New York City has invested in the procedural-justice approach by promoting its use in the city court system, providing training to criminal court personnel, and redesigning courthouse décor and architecture.

New York City's approach to crime and violence prevention has paid big dividends in decreasing the number of crimes and reducing the jail population, and for these reasons, the city's approach is often held up as a model for other cities. However, what works in one city may not work in another, and a trial-and-error strategy is needed to see what is effective and what is not for a particular urban setting. This explains why a multifaceted crime prevention strategy is needed, where the successful elements can be retained while less successful elements are discarded. Crime and violence remain high in some parts of New York City, and city officials know that they cannot let their guard down, but the successes achieved to date are fostering optimism about preventing a return to the days when crime in the city was rampant.

Drugs and Alcohol

The abuse of drugs and alcohol is one of the most serious public health problems in the United States and many other countries, affecting rich and poor alike and showing no preference for any ethnic or social groups. Most people who abuse drugs and alcohol are productive members of society with jobs and families, who often believe that their drug or alcohol use is under control. However, for many individuals, drug and alcohol abuse tends to worsen over time, eventually disrupting their normal routines and causing anguish among family, friends, and coworkers. A parent's drug or alcohol problems can be particularly damaging to young children and adolescents, who look up to their parents as role models and sometimes experience domestic violence associated with drug or alcohol abuse.

The effects of drug and alcohol abuse on a global scale are staggering. The World Health Organization (WHO) reports that globally, the harmful use of alcohol alone causes over 3 million deaths every year, with high-income countries having the highest alcohol-per-capita consumption rates and highest prevalence of heavy episodic drinking. In the United States, about 90,000 people die annually from alcohol-related causes, making it the third-leading preventable cause of death (after tobacco use, and poor diet combined with physical inactivity), and drug overdoses cause over 70,000 American deaths annually, as illustrated in Figure 2. The highest drug-related mortality rate in the world is in North America (i.e., the United States and Canada), which accounts for one in four drug deaths globally. The abuse of tobacco, alcohol, and illicit drugs in the United States alone results in over $700 billion per year in costs associated with healthcare, crime, and lost productivity. With over half of the world's population living in urban areas, the challenges faced by many cities in addressing drug and alcohol problems cannot be overstated.

The use of mind-altering substances has been around for a long time, probably throughout much of human history. Drugs and alcohol were used by ancient civilizations for religious practices, and this use continues today in some cultures. Drug and alcohol abuse may begin with experimentation, social use, and self-medication (e.g., attempts at relieving chronic pain), and coping with loneliness and depression also can lead to abuse for some people. All ages can be affected, from childhood and adolescence through old age. While drug and alcohol abuse is widespread, it is particularly a problem in many urban areas due to the ease of acquiring these substances by people struggling with the stresses of modern city life. Additionally, the deteriorating social-cultural environment in some high-crime city neighborhoods can push local residents toward excessive drug and alcohol use.

The term "drug" is a generic reference to a variety of prescription, nonprescription, and illicit substances, some of which can affect behavior and potentially become addictive. Alcohol is a drug, along with the nicotine in

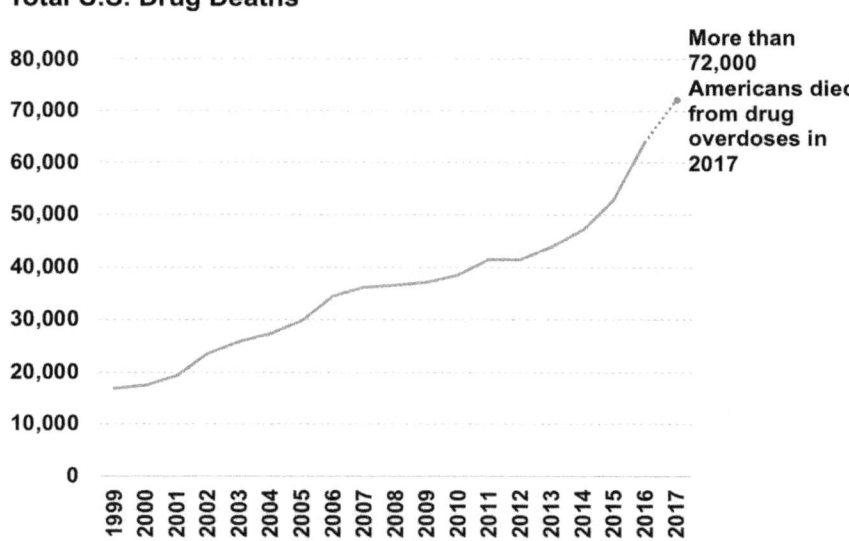

Figure 2   Deaths in the United States from drug overdoses, including illicit drugs and prescription opioids. (*Source:* National Institute on Drug Abuse.)

tobacco products and the caffeine in beverages like coffee. Many drugs are lifesaving, some drugs have adverse side effects, and other drugs can be abused. The use of the term "drugs and alcohol" here generally refers to substances with the potential to be abused and which are not used for beneficial medical reasons, except where medical drugs are taken in excess or used for other than their intended purposes. Table 7 presents descriptions of common legal and illegal drugs and controlled substances (i.e., drugs declared illegal for sale or use, but which may be dispensed under a physician's prescription).

Understanding the hazards associated with drug and alcohol abuse and addiction can be complicated because various agencies and organizations use inconsistent terminology to describe different forms and degrees of abuse and addiction. The leading U.S. agency that deals with drug abuse, the National Institute of Drug Abuse (NIDA), has defined "drug abuse" and "addiction" this way:

> People use substances for a variety of reasons. It becomes drug abuse when people use illegal drugs or use legal drugs inappropriately. This includes the repeated use of drugs to produce pleasure, alleviate stress, and/or alter or avoid reality. It also includes using prescription drugs in ways other than prescribed or using someone else's prescription. Addiction occurs when a person cannot control the impulse to use drugs even when there are negative consequences—the defining characteristic of addiction. These behavioral changes are also accompanied by changes in brain functioning, especially in the brain's natural inhibition and reward centers. NIDA's use of the term addiction corresponds roughly to the DSM [Diagnostic and Statistical Manual of Mental Disorders] definition of substance use disorder. The DSM does not use the term addiction.

Thus, drug abuse (also called "substance abuse") involves the use of illegal drugs or the use of legal drugs inappropriately (e.g., to produce pleasure, alleviate stress, or avoid reality), whereas drug addiction (roughly corresponding to the term "substance use disorder") occurs when a person cannot resist the impulse to use drugs even where there are negative consequences. You can think of abuse as an early stage of addiction—as abuse becomes more frequent, the likelihood of becoming addicted becomes greater. Recently, the NIDA has begun using the term "misuse" in place of "abuse" in many of its publications, noting that the terms are "roughly equivalent." According to the NIDA, "'Substance abuse' is a

Table 7   Common Legal and Illegal Drugs and Controlled Substances

Category	Description
LEGAL DRUGS	
Alcohol	Alcohol is the top drug that is abused in the United States, and alcoholism is a serious problem worldwide. Binge drinking (five or more drinks on a single occasion for men, and four or more for women) by high school and college students, usually involving beer, is especially concerning. Alcohol consumption contributes to automobile accidents, violence (e.g., child abuse, sexual assault, homicide, suicide, spouse or partner abuse, and vandalism), and unintentional injuries and deaths (e.g., drowning, falling, and burns).
Nicotine	This is the psychoactive and addictive drug found in tobacco products, such as cigarettes, cigars, and chewing and pipe tobacco. Smoking is associated with respiratory and cardiovascular disease and with cancer that can occur almost anywhere in the body. In the United States, cigarette smoking is the leading preventable cause of death.
Prescription and over-the-counter pharmaceuticals	These pharmaceuticals are ordinarily safe when prescription or label instructions are followed, although unwanted side effects can occur with some products. Drug misuse occurs when taking more or less than the amount prescribed or instructed (either intentionally or unintentionally), and drug abuse occurs when using pharmaceuticals for other than their intended purpose. Misuse or abuse of pharmaceuticals can lead to dependency, risk of injury of death from overdose, and development of drug-resistant strains of pathogens.

(continued)

Table 7   (continued)

Category	Description

ILLEGAL DRUGS AND CONTROLLED SUBSTANCES

Category	Description
Anabolic drugs	These protein-building drugs (e.g., anabolic/ androgenic steroids, testosterone, and human growth hormone) are sometimes abused by athletes and bodybuilders to increase muscle mass, strength, and endurance rapidly. Abuse of these drugs can lead to a number of unwanted side effects, and long-term abuse can result in psychological dependency.
Club and designer drugs	"Club drugs" are primarily drugs most commonly used in nightclubs and bars and at parties, and they are often taken in combination with other drugs and alcohol. One of the more popular club drugs, 3,4-met hylenedioxymethamphetamine (MDMA, also known as ecstasy), produces an energizing effect, distorts time and perception, and enhances sensory experiences. Another club drug, D-lysergic acid diethylamide (LSD, also known as "acid," "blotter," "dots," and "yellow sunshine") is one of the most powerful mood-changing chemicals. The term "designer drugs" refers to various drugs synthesized by amateur chemists, often changing formulas to escape detection by law enforcement. Examples include MDMA, synthetic narcotics, ketamine (also known as "K," "special K," or "cat valium"), and phencyclidine (PCP; also known as "angel dust," "hog," "love boat," and "peace pill").
Cocaine	Cocaine (also called "coca," "coke," "crack," "flake," "snow," and "soda cot") is a stimulant, derived from the leaves of coca plants, that increases activity in the central nervous system. In its purer form as a salt (appearing as a white powder) or dried paste (called "crack"), it becomes a highly addictive and potent euphoriant. Other effects include increased alertness and excitation, restlessness, irritability, and anxiety, and taking

Table 7   (continued)

Category	Description
	high doses or using over prolonged periods usually causes paranoia. Because tolerance to cocaine develops rapidly, users require higher and higher doses to satisfy their craving.
Depressants	Depressants include barbiturates, benzodiazapines, and methaqualone. Their effect is to slow down the nervous system, which can initially lower anxiety and reduce inhabitation. But tolerance develops with continued use, resulting in higher and higher doses and eventually a strong dependence, requiring medical intervention for detoxification and recovery.
Hallucinogens	These drugs cause illusions, hallucinations, and other perception changes due to synesthesia, which is the brain's mixing of the senses. Examples of hallucinogens are mescaline (derived from the peyote cactus), psilocybin and psilocin (derived from the *Psilocybe* mushroom), and LSD (a synthetic drug).
Inhalants	This term refers to a variety of inhalable chemicals that often act as depressants, reducing anxieties and inhibitions, and with continued use, causing hallucinations and loss of consciousness. Examples are paint solvents, motor fuels, cleaners, glues, aerosol sprays, and cosmetics. These chemicals can be extremely toxic to the kidneys, liver, and nervous system.
Marijuana	Marijuana (also called "weed," "pot," "dope," and "cannabis") is derived from the hemp plant, and it is illegal in many countries, including the United States, where use continues to be prohibited under federal law. However, a number of states have challenged the federal law by enacted legislation legalizing marijuana for medical use and in some cases

(continued)

Table 7   (continued)

Category	Description
	recreational use. Additionally, some states have decriminalized the possession of small amounts. Among its medical uses, marijuana may help prevent and ease nausea caused by chemotherapy, treat chronic pain (reducing the initial need for opioids), and ease opioid withdrawal symptoms, and there is evidence that it can help heal the diseased addict's brain as well. The U.S. Centers for Disease Control and Prevention (CDC) reports on a number of potential adverse side effects of marijuana use (cdc.gov/marijuana), including addiction affecting about one in ten marijuana users (one in six users if use began before age 18), lung tissue damage and and a greater risk of cough and bronchitis if smoked, unpleasant thoughts or feelings of anxiety and paranoia if used frequently or in high doses, and adverse effects on brain development, particularly when users begin as teenagers.
Narcotics	Also known as "opioids," narcotics are a class of drugs that dull the senses and relieve pain. Examples are heroin and pharmaceutical drugs like OxyContin, Vicodin, codeine, morphine, methadone, and fentanyl. Narcotics produce euphoria, analgesia, and drowsiness and reduce anxiety, making them ideal candidates for abuse. Because the body develops a tolerance to narcotics, larger and larger doses are required to achieve the same effects as the initial dose. This makes narcotic addiction particularly dangerous. According to the CDC, opioid misuse and addiction in the United States is a serious national crisis, causing over 115 overdose deaths every day.

Table 7   (continued)

Category	Description
Stimulants	Stimulants increase activity in the central system by causing release of the neurotransmitter dopamine. Examples are amphetamine (known as "bennies"), dextroamphetamine ("dexies"), methamphetamine ("meth," "crystal," "crank," "speed," or "go fast"), dextromethamphetamine ("ice"), methcathinone ("cat"), and methylphenidate (Ritalin, a drug used to treat attention deficit hyperactivity disorder). Users must increase doses because tolerance builds up quickly, and long-term effects of repeated use can include memory loss and brain damage.

Sources: J. F. McKenzie and R. R. Pringer, *An Introduction to Community and Public Health,* Jones and Bartlett Learning, Burlington (2015); Centers for Disease Control and Prevention (CDC); Drug Enforcement Administration (DEA); National Institute on Drug Abuse (NIDA).

diagnostic term that is increasingly avoided by professionals because it can be shaming, and adds to the stigma that often keeps people from asking for help. 'Substance misuse' suggests use that can cause harm to the user or their friends or family." Other organizations clarify that "misuse" is specifically when a prescription drug is used for a purpose other than its intended purpose, while still other organizations have been reluctant to use this terminology at all. The use of differing terminology in the United States and throughout the world sometimes complicates conversations about drugs and alcohol, leading to misunderstandings.

The NIDA has defined another key term, "physical dependence," as follows:

Physical dependence can happen with the chronic use of many drugs—including many prescription drugs, even if taken as instructed. Thus, physical dependence in and of itself does not constitute addiction, but it often accompanies addiction. This distinction can be difficult to discern, particularly with prescribed pain medications, for which the need for increasing dosages can represent tolerance or a worsening underlying problem, as opposed to the beginning of abuse or addiction.

In contrast to physical dependence, mental dependence occurs when the use of a substance is a conditioned response to events or feelings, which are known as "triggers." Addiction usually involves both physical and mental dependence. Other terms to be familiar with are:

- **Denial**—when drug users do not believe they have a problem despite strong evidence to the contrary
- **Detoxifiation**—a process that helps rid the body of harmful substances while withdrawal symptoms are being treated
- **Relapse**—the recurrence of symptoms (e.g., when a person in recovery cannot resist the urge to drink or use drugs again after a period of abstinence)
- **Treatment plan**—a plan developed with the assistance of health-care professionals that describes the addiction problem, treatment goals, and specific steps to be followed by treatment professionals and the patient
- **Trigger**—something like an event, place, item, smell, idea, emotion, or person that causes a craving to use drugs or drink alcohol

Nearly all addictive drugs, including alcohol, cause the release of increased levels of dopamine, a neurotransmitter in the brain that regulates movement, emotion, cognition, motivation, and feelings of pleasure. This extra dopamine produces euphoric effects that cause users to continue using the drugs to satisfy their cravings. Drug use is initially voluntary, but it becomes involuntary in addicts when they lose their ability for self-control and become seriously impaired, resulting in compulsive and sometimes destructive behaviors. In people suffering from drug and alcohol addiction, there are changes to the structure of the brain, particularly to the brain's natural inhibition and reward centers. Thus, drug addiction is considered a chronic brain disease, characterized by compulsive drug-seeking and use despite the harmful consequences.

Some people are more at risk for drug and alcohol abuse than others. A number of studies indicate that a predisposition to alcoholism can be inherited, and there is some evidence that genes may also play a role in cigarette smoking. Personality can be a factor in drug and alcohol abuse, such as whether someone is impulsive and willing to take chances, and environmental factors can also play a role, such as issues with family or work life and the social-cultural environment in which one lives. Product advertising, including ads aimed at adolescents, can have a big influence on alcohol consumption and cigarette smoking.

Teens and college students are often considered more susceptible to drug and alcohol abuse than postcollege adults because younger people are more likely to experiment with drugs and alcohol and to be influenced to do so by peer pressure. Older adults are also more susceptible because they are more likely to have high blood pressure, diabetes, arthritis, or some other chronic medical disorder requiring medication, and they may be taking other drugs on a short-term basis for acute issues, such as infections, general aches and pains, and constipation. Nearly half of adults age 65 and older take at least five different pharmaceuticals every week, and nursing home patients take, on average, between seven and eight different drugs weekly. As these multiple drugs build up in a person's system, the possibility of adverse interactions among drugs increases, causing added concern for dependence and addiction. In addition to seeking relief from physical ailments, some older adults turn to drugs to help cope with loneliness and depression.

IMPACT ON URBAN HEALTH

Drug and alcohol problems are rife within the city, and in many major metropolitan areas, hardly a day goes by without news of a drug-related death or alcohol-related freeway accident. Gang and domestic violence related to drugs and alcohol are also frequently reported. The risks to health of drug addiction and alcohol abuse are well known, particularly destructive changes in behavior and mental acuity that can compromise health and sometimes result in prolonged treatment, hospitalization, and even death. Also, infections among people who use drugs are common, including HIV/ AIDS, hepatitis, sexually transmitted diseases, and tuberculosis. Destructive binge drinking (five or more drinks on a single occasion for males, and four or more for females) has been on the rise, particularly affecting inner-city and suburban high school and college students.

In addition to the physical and mental issues surrounding drug and alcohol abuse, the consequences can include the following:

- arrest for criminal activity
- financial instability
- increased motor vehicle accidents

- loss of employment
- marriage and other family problems
- missed days from school or work
- problems staying in school or keeping a job
- suicide

Families can also suffer from turmoil and financial strain when a family member abuses drugs or alcohol, and family members can become depressed themselves, requiring medical attention. Drug and alcohol-related domestic violence and broken homes are unfortunately all too common in the city, and neighborhoods trying to cope with increased drug-related illness and violence may become overwhelmed as they set up drug treatment programs while addressing the spread of sexually transmitted diseases and increased emergency room admissions.

Many cities in the United States and other nations are experiencing what is termed an "opioid crisis" involving the misuse and abuse of prescription opioids, such as hydrocodone, oxycodone, morphine, and codeine, and the illegal opioid, heroin. Opioids have historically been used as painkillers, and they have great potential for misuse due to their common availability for medical purposes. According to the CDC, 115 Americans die every day from an opioid overdose, and from 1999 to 2016, there were over 350,000 opioid overdose deaths. It is believed that about half of people misusing prescription painkillers get them from friends or relatives, and nearly 25 percent receive them from a doctor. With repeated use of opioids, people's tolerance for the drugs increases, resulting in the desire for higher and higher doses to achieve the same effect and avoid withdrawal. As individuals require more drugs, they sometimes turn to the black market, switching to cheaper and riskier substitutes for prescription opioids, like heroin.

According to the National Survey on Drug Use and Health, over 4 million Americans are engaged in nonmedical use of prescription painkillers every month, and nearly 5 million Americans have used heroin at some point in their lives. Nonaddictive painkillers currently under development show promise for relieving pain without the risk of opioid addiction. However, clinical trials spanning multiple years are needed to determine whether the painkillers are safe and effective and to what extent they can be used under a variety of scenarios involving pain.

While emphasizing that drinking too much can cause a range of consequences and increase risk for a variety of problems, the National Institute on Alcohol Abuse and Alcoholism notes that "moderate alcohol consumption may have beneficial effects on health. These include decreased risk for heart disease and mortality due to heart disease, decreased risk of ischemic stroke (in which the arteries to the brain become narrowed or blocked, resulting in reduced blood flow), and decreased risk of diabetes." The key term here is *moderate* alcohol consumption. The 2015–2020 Dietary Guidelines for Americans cautions that "if alcohol is consumed, it should be in moderation—up to one drink per day for women and up to two drinks per day for men—and only by adults of legal drinking age. For those who choose to drink, moderate alcohol consumption can be incorporated into the calorie limits of most healthy eating patterns. The Dietary Guidelines does not recommend that individuals who do not drink alcohol start drinking for any reason; however, it does recommend that all foods and beverages consumed be accounted for within healthy eating patterns."

WHAT CITIES ARE DOING ABOUT DRUGS AND ALCOHOL

While a variety of drug and alcohol abuse prevention and control programs are available at the state and federal levels of government, it has become increasing obvious that the war on drugs is most successful at the local level, within our cities, neighborhoods, homes, and schools. Many communities have prevention and control programs in place across a number of agencies and offices, such as health departments, the juvenile justice system and courts, police departments, and family services offices. And often drug task forces are formed, made up of community leaders, health experts, social workers, and educators who coordinate efforts across the city and design strategies that can be most effective for the drug problems unique to their particular locale.

Cities have also implemented special taxes to discourage alcohol and tobacco use, zoning ordinances in high-crime areas to limit the number of bars and liquor stores, and beefed-up police patrols to catch drug offenders. While these initiatives have been effective, many public health professionals believe that a more enlightened approach to solving the drug and alcohol crisis—creating job opportunities, improving education and housing, expanding social services, and providing free or affordable healthcare—will ultimately be needed for long-term success. Additionally, some experts believe that faith groups can play an important role through counseling and worship.

Nongovernmental programs in urban areas have also been very effective in educating the public about drug abuse prevention and control and providing culturally sensitive, multilingual programs to help abusers and their loved ones cope with drug abuse problems at home. Many successful programs are school based, such as the Drug Abuse Resistance Education (DARE), a police officer–led series of classroom lessons that teaches children from kindergarten through 12th grade how to resist peer pressure and live drug- and violence-free lives. DARE envisions "a world in which students everywhere are empowered to respect others and choose to lead lives free from violence, substance abuse, and other dangerous behaviors." Other well-known and successful programs that are national in scope and implemented locally include Alcoholics Anonymous (AA), Mothers Against Drunk Driving (MADD), and Students Against Destructive Decisions (SADD).

Within school systems, peer counseling can also be effective in preventing drug and alcohol abuse. Peer counseling occurs when students share problems among themselves in a safe, nonjudgmental environment, helping each other cope with abuse and addiction involving themselves, their friends, or loved ones at home. Often, peers trained in intervention participate in or lead peer-counseling sessions.

Unfortunately, drug and alcohol abuse can be a serious problem in the workplace, resulting in absenteeism, reduced productivity, and even risk of serious injury where heavy equipment and machinery is involved, and drug and alcohol abuse also can lead to workplace violence. As a result, many companies have implemented programs aimed at employee drug education and awareness, supervisor training, and employee assistance for workers needing counseling and rehabilitation. Additionally, drug testing (i.e., screening for drugs, such as amphetamines, cocaine, marijuana, opioids, and phencyclidine) has been implemented at many companies as new workers are brought on board, and occasionally for existing employees as well, particularly if the employees are involved in jobs posing a significant safety risk to themselves or others. (A positive drug test or history of drug use or abuse can be cause for rejecting applicants or dismissing current workers.) In the United States, the Drug-Free Federal Workplace program is designed to address illicit drug use where federal employees are involved.

RECOMMENDATIONS FOR CITY DWELLERS

Drug abuse is a serious issue that, left untreated, can lead to drug dependence and alcoholism. Thus, it is important to be able to recognize the symptoms of drug abuse among friends and family members, as well as in yourself. By recognizing the symptoms early, it is much easier to avoid more serious problems farther down the road.

Symptoms associated with alcohol use disorder include:

- Temporary blackouts or memory loss
- Recurrent arguments or fights with family members or friends, as well as irritability, depression, or mood swings
- Continuing use of alcohol to relax, cheer up, sleep, deal with problems, or feel "normal"
- Headache, anxiety, insomnia, nausea, or other unpleasant symptoms when one stops drinking
- Flushed skin and broken capillaries on the face, a husky voice, trembling hands, bloody or black/tarry stools, chronic diarrhea, or vomiting blood
- Drinking alone, in the mornings or in secret

Signs of drug and alcohol addiction include:

- Loss of control—drinking or drugging more than people want to, for longer than they intended, or despite telling themselves that they "wouldn't do it this time"
- Neglecting other activities—spending less time on activities that used to be important (hanging out with family and friends, exercising, pursuing hobbies or other interests) because of using alcohol or drugs; drops in attendance or performance at work or school
- Risk taking—more likely to take serious risks in order to obtain one's drug of choice
- Relationship issues—people struggling with addiction acting out against those closest to them, particularly if they are attempting to address their substance problems; complaints from coworkers, supervisors, teachers, or classmates
- Secrecy—going out of one's way to hide the amount of drugs or alcohol consumed or one's activities when drinking or drugging; unexplained injuries or accidents

- Changing appearance—serious changes or deterioration in hygiene or physical appearance, including lack of showering, slovenly appearance, unclean clothes
- Family history—a family history of addiction can dramatically increase one's predisposition to substance abuse
- Tolerance—over time, a person's body adapting to a substance to the point that they need more and more of it in order to have the same reaction
- Withdrawal—as the effect of the alcohol or drugs wear off, experiencing symptoms such as anxiety or jumpiness, shakiness or trembling, sweating, nausea and vomiting, insomnia, depression, irritability, fatigue or loss of appetite, and headaches
- Continued use despite negative consequences—drinking or drugging even though it is causing problems (on the job, in relationships, for one's health)

Remember that denial—believing that you do not have a drug or alcohol problem despite strong evidence to the contrary—is common among people with use and abuse problems. Thus, if you experience any symptoms of abuse and addiction, you should seek help even if you do not think you need it. If you are a young person, you are especially at risk. Table 8 presents 10 tips that young people can follow to prevent drug abuse.

An important resource for information and assistance is the Substance Abuse and Mental Health Services Administration (SAMHSA) National Helpline [800-662-HELP (4357)], also known as the Treatment Referral Routing Service. This is a confidential, free, 24-hour information service in English and Spanish for individuals and family members facing mental or substance use disorders. The service provides referrals to local treatment facilities, support groups, and community-based organizations, and callers can also order free publications and other information. Attesting to the popularity of the National Helpline, the service has been receiving over 800,000 calls annually. Also, do not hesitate to use the National Suicide Prevention Lifeline (800-273-TALK, or 800-273-8255) or to refer friends to it.

Table 8   10 Tips for Youths for Preventing Drug and Alcohol Problems

Tips for Prevention	Main Points
1. Don't be afraid to say no.	Sometimes our fear of negative reaction from our friends, or people we don't even know, keeps us from doing what we know is right. It's really simple—it may seem like "everyone is doing it," but they are not. Don't let someone else make your decisions for you. If someone is pressuring you to do something that's not right for you, you have the right to say no, the right not to give a reason why, and the right to just walk away.
2. Connect with your friends and avoid negative peer pressure.	Pay attention to the people you are hanging out with. If you are hanging out with a group in which the majority of kids are drinking alcohol or using drugs to get high, you may want to think about making some new friends. You may be headed toward an alcohol and drug problem if you continue to hang around others who routinely drink alcohol, smoke marijuana, abuse prescription drugs, or use illegal drugs. You don't have to go along to get along.
3. Make connections with your parents or other adults.	As you grow up, having people you can rely on—people you can talk to about life, life's challenges, and your decisions about alcohol and drugs—is very important. The opportunity to benefit from someone else's life experiences can help put things in perspective and can be invaluable.
4. Enjoy life and do what you love—don't add alcohol and drugs.	Learn how to enjoy life and the people in your life without adding alcohol or drugs. Alcohol and drugs can change who you are, limit your potential, and complicate your life. Too often, "I'm bored" is just an excuse. Get out and get active in school and community activities such as music, sports, arts, or a part-time job. Giving back as a volunteer is a great way to gain perspective on life.

(*continued*)

Table 8   (continued)

Tips for Prevention	Main Points
5. Follow the family rules about alcohol and drugs.	As you grow up and want to assume more control over your life, having the trust and respect of your parents is very important. Don't let alcohol and drugs come between you and your parents. Talking with your mom and dad about alcohol and drugs can be very helpful.
6. Get educated about alcohol and drugs.	You cannot rely on the myths and misconceptions that are out there among your friends and on the internet. Your ability to make the right decisions includes getting educated. Visit the "Facts About Alcohol" and "Facts About Drugs" pages at the National Council on Alcoholism and Drug Dependence website (ncadd.org). And, as you learn, share what you are learning with your friends and your family.
7. Be a role model and set a positive example.	Don't forget—what you do is more important than what you say! You are setting the foundation of and the direction for your life; where are you headed?
8. Plan ahead.	As you make plans for a party or going out with friends, you need to plan ahead. You need to protect yourself and be smart. Don't become a victim of someone else's alcohol or drug use. Make sure that there is someone you can call (day or night, no matter what) if you need them. And do the same for your friends.
9. Speak out/ speak up/take control.	Take responsibility for your life, your health, and your safety. Speak up about what alcohol and drugs are doing to your friends and your community, and encourage others to do the same.
10. Get help!	If you or someone you know is in trouble with alcohol or drugs, get help. Don't wait. You don't have to be alone.

Source: National Council on Alcoholism and Drug Dependence.

EXPERT COMMENTARY: SUBSTANCE AVAILABILITY AND ABUSE

Treatment needs have perpetually outweighed availability of services in urban areas, and lack of funding is another persistent problem.

Victor B. Stolberg, Assistant Professor/Counselor

Essex County College

Victor Stolberg is an assistant professor/counselor at Essex County College in Newark, New Jersey. He has served there for over three decades, previously directing both the Office of the Substance Abuse Coordinator and the Office of Disability Support Services. Prior to this, Professor Stolberg helped develop the Alcohol Awareness Program at the University of Buffalo. He has written hundreds of scholarly articles, chapters, and encyclopedia entries and served on various boards, including the editorial board of the Journal of Ethnicity in Substance Abuse. *Additionally, Professor Stolberg has written the following books:* Painkillers: History, Science, and Issues; ADHD Medications: History, Science, and Issues; *and* What You Need to Know About ADHD.

What do you see as the greatest issues regarding substance availability and abuse in urban areas, what are the major obstacles to addressing these issues, and what is your hope for the future?

The factors affecting substance abuse in urban areas are reflective of those impacting urban residents generally. Urban centers are by definition densely populated geographic spaces, which generate a particular set of deep concerns, such as poverty, racism, and violence, but unfortunately, there is generally not a concomitant array of services provided.

According to SAMHSA, urban substance users differ from their rural counterparts in several crucial areas. Urban users are less likely to abuse alcohol, 36.1 percent compared to 49.5 percent, but more likely to abuse traditional street drugs, such as heroin and cocaine. While 21.8 percent of urban users report heroin as their drug of choice, only 3.1 percent of rural users do. Similarly, 11.9 percent of urban users report cocaine as their drug of choice, compared to 5.6 percent of rural users. Unfortunately, urban users are less likely to be court ordered into treatment, 28.4 percent compared to 51.6 percent for rural peers. Treatment needs have perpetually outweighed availability of services in urban areas, and lack of funding is another persistent problem. On a brighter note, urban residents are more likely to enter treatment voluntarily or under pressure from family members. Users entering treatment in urban areas are more ethnically diverse and tend to have lower levels of education and higher rates of unemployment.

The very strong positive relationship between availability and abuse has been observed time and again with many different substances, including alcohol, tobacco, cocaine, and opiates, and it would be no surprise when looking more closely at urban areas that such has been the case for many other substances. In this regard, I sincerely hope that the emerging trends toward decriminalization and legalization of recreational use of cannabis by states and municipalities can be curtailed and reversed. Such measures run contrary to what we have learned about the effective prevention of substance abuse problems, particularly the importance of maintaining clear, broad-based, consistent approaches. Otherwise, given our understandings of substances, we can expect a wave of adverse unintended effects from increased cannabis use, including in already strained urban areas.

Urban users face myriad structural problems, such as residential segregation, neighborhood deprivation, family fragmentation, and inequitable income distribution. Until some of these fundamental issues are more comprehensively addressed, substance use is likely to remain symptomatic of the broader challenges facing urban residents. However, should we rise to the challenges, then great strides can be expected in the future.

Food Quality and Availability

From the beginning of human existence, daily activities have revolved around obtaining food, and every culture has developed traditions regarding food preparation and consumption. Today, maintaining access to quality food sources is a critical part of governance, and threats to urban health often result when food quality and availability are compromised.

When city dwellers have an inadequate diet due to poverty or the effects of drug or alcohol abuse, poor nutrition can make them more susceptible to disease and mental distress. To prevent nutritional deficiencies and encourage a healthy diet, nutritionists often discuss the nutritional content of food in terms of micronutrients and macronutrients. "Micronutrients" are the vitamins and minerals that people need only in small amounts, although consuming enough micronutrients is essential because they are critical building blocks for the proteins and hormones required for proper bodily function. Deficiencies in the micronutrients iodine, vitamin A, and iron are important global health concerns because they are associated with various health problems in low- and middle-income countries, including blindness, mental impairment, and anemia.

In contrast to micronutrients, "macronutrients" are the fats, carbohydrates, and proteins that people need to eat in relatively large amounts. Consuming too few macronutrients can cause growth and developmental problems, especially in children, but eating too many can cause obesity and related diseases, such as heart disease and diabetes. Obesity-related diseases are widespread in the United States, where over one-third of the adult population (nearly 100 million people) is considered obese. Worldwide, nearly 40 percent of adults are overweight or obese, contributing to at least 2.8 million deaths annually. Obesity, once associated only with affluent, developed nations, is now prevalent in low- and middle-income countries as well, possibly because processed, low-quality foods high in fats and sugars are often cheap and readily available.

In the city, many healthy food options are available that deliver more than enough micronutrients and macronutrients, especially for residents who can afford to shop at specialty grocery stores or the local farmers' market. However, because of busy work and family schedules and long commutes, many city residents choose to eat out regularly, including grabbing a sandwich at a fast-food restaurant, rather than cooking healthy meals at home. A recent Gallop poll found that nearly a quarter of Americans eat dinner at restaurants two times a week, and another quarter eat dinner out three or more times a week, and in addition, many are eating out for breakfast and lunch. Eating away from home can also be expensive. For example, residents of the New York City area spend nearly $3,000 per year on food away from home, representing about 44 percent of their total food budget, according to the U.S. Bureau of Labor Statistics.

To help people make good dietary choices, many countries, including the United States, have developed food guides describing the amounts and types of foods that people should eat. These guides often focus on the major food groups—grains, dairy, fruits, and vegetables—and are illustrated by shapes that visually represent suggested proportions for a good diet. Most Americans are familiar with the food pyramid and newer MyPlate representation, illustrating the proportion of each food group that should be present in a healthy diet. Other countries use shapes that are culturally significant, like the spinning top that Japan uses for its food guide.

Foodborne diseases are often caused by improper food handling and storage, either at the farm, during transportation, or during meal preparation. A recent example of a nationwide foodborne disease occurrence is the 2018 *Escherichia coli* outbreak caused by eating lettuce from the Yuma, Arizona, area. The Centers for Disease Control and Prevention (CDC) reports that 210 people in 36 states who had eaten that lettuce were infected with a particularly virulent strain of *E. coli* that can cause cramps, bloody diarrhea, and even kidney failure and death. (According to the CDC, 96 people were hospitalized, including 27 with kidney failure, and 5 of them died.) The outbreak, which was traced to tainted irrigation water from a canal in the Yuma area, was the largest U.S. outbreak of *E. coli* in more than a decade. Previously, the largest *E. coli* outbreak involved spinach grown in California in 2006, which was probably contaminated by wild pigs roaming through a stream infested with *E. coli* and then spreading the bacteria to nearby spinach fields.

As city populations grow, maintaining a safe and healthy food supply becomes a larger issue, especially in urban areas that rely on rural farms to provide fresh food. Threats to the urban food supply include weather-based damage to the food crops, the introduction of foodborne pathogens, and inefficient food distribution networks. Providing an adequate food supply to urban areas, particularly for families with limited resources, may become even more challenging in the future as climate change worsens, social inequalities grow, and urban farms increasingly face extinction due to a variety of environmental and economic stressors. Providing a sustainable food supply for the entire global population may be one of the greatest challenges of the twenty-first century.

IMPACT ON URBAN HEALTH

The contamination of food with toxins or pathogens (agents of infection and disease) poses a significant threat to food quality in urban areas, particularly in parts of the world where food quality is compromised by lack of refrigeration and inefficient distribution networks. The most common foodborne pathogens include *Norovirus*, *Salmonella*, and *Staphylococcus aureus*. Typically, the illnesses caused by these pathogens result in nausea, vomiting, stomach cramps, and diarrhea within hours or days of ingesting the contaminated food. Other foodborne pathogens, which are less common but more likely to cause hospitalization, are *E. coli*, *Listeria*, and *Clostridium botulinum* (the causative agent of botulism).

Food selection choices can also have a negative impact on the diet of individuals in cities. Income-based health disparities in the United States and many other countries are associated, in part, with the food choices made by people of differing socioeconomic status. This difference in food choice has been attributed to a number of factors, including the relatively higher cost of fresh foods, insufficient education about good nutritional habits, and the presence of food deserts in low-income areas. "Food deserts" are areas altogether lacking stores that carry fresh foods. This restricts residents without cars to grocery shopping in convenience stores, which typically do not carry the fresh fruits and vegetables required for a healthy diet, and instead sell high-fat, highly processed foods that often contribute to obesity.

Food deserts are predominantly found in low-income urban areas, and many public health researchers attribute income-based health disparities to reduced access to nutritious foods in these areas. This lack of food options also makes impoverished individuals living in urban areas more susceptible to foodborne diseases and other threats to public health. However, food deserts alone do not explain the disparity between the eating choices made by low- and high-income families. One study found that when new supermarkets were opened in food deserts, local families continued to buy food of the same nutritional value, despite the greater availability of fresh food. Other studies have found that increased education about good nutrition, in conjunction with access to fresh, wholesome food, is required to improve eating habits.

Future access to healthy food may become more difficult due to the effects of climate change—crop damage from extreme weather conditions, increased insect infestations, and the inundation of coastal farmlands from rising sea levels. Other environmental threats to farmland include water pollution, reduced groundwater supply, and depletion of soil nutrients due to high-volume farming practices. As urban areas encroach on rural farmlands, farm production is under further threat—agricultural lands the size of Italy will be lost to increased global urbanization within the next 20 years.

WHAT CITIES ARE DOING ABOUT FOOD QUALITY AND AVAILABILITY

City governments, usually through their public health departments, are on the frontline of ensuring food safety and preventing foodborne illnesses. Specifically, city inspectors visit retail food outlets, such as restaurants and grocery stores, to ensure that they are following safe food-handling procedures and to enforce remedial actions when violations are found. How often these inspections occur and what they include are determined by local laws and regulations, but typically, the inspectors assess whether appropriate safeguards are in place to prevent food contamination (e.g., from contact with unclean food-handling equipment or surfaces or from inadequate preparation techniques). In the United States, cities often coordinate food safety concerns with state and federal agencies, including the Department of Agriculture (USDA), the Food and Drug Administration (FDA), and the CDC. For example, the USDA regulates and monitors farm production of food, the FDA enforces food labeling regulations and issues food recalls, and the CDC investigates disease outbreaks related to contaminated food and issues warnings to the public.

Food waste is a big problem in American cities. The USDA estimates that between 30 and 40 percent of the food supply is wasted, which has far-reaching effects on the U.S. economy and the environment. Much of this food waste could be used to feed families in need, and the environmental impacts from growing, processing, transporting, preparing, storing, and disposing of food that is ultimately wasted may "endanger the long-run health of the planet," according to the USDA. Furthermore, food waste is the largest component of municipal landfills, and as such, is responsible for vast emissions of methane, a potent greenhouse gas (GHG).

To address the food waste problem, a number of cities have programs aimed at reducing food waste at home and restaurants, and many grocery stores and restaurants offer unused food to homeless shelters and other non-profit organizations. To reduce wastes going to landfills, it is increasingly common for urban areas to encourage or require the composting of organic waste. Some cities maintain large municipal composting facilities, and many homeowners compost at home.

Along with reducing food waste, many cities are improving urban access to fresh food by developing community gardens, which are plots of land used by local residents for communal gardening. Community gardens are typically owned by a city or a nonprofit organization and managed by people living in the surrounding area. These gardens come in all shapes and sizes, from large plots used to grow vegetables for local residents and low-income families to small planters on street corners tended by individuals. Some cities encourage community gardens by providing instructional guides, gardening expertise, and grants to nonprofits.

Community gardens shorten the food supply chain by generating local food for urban dwellers. In addition to making the food supply safer by eliminating many potential sources of contamination, shortening the path from farm to table also limits the environmental footprint of food by reducing the use of large farm machinery and eliminating the need for produce to be shipped to a city. Working in a community garden can benefit people's health by providing exercise and access to fresh fruit and vegetables, and mental health is also improved by creating a healthy social activity and creating local green space.

To ensure that low-income children have access to healthy, balanced meals, many city public and nonprofit private schools and residential child-care institutions in the United States participate in school breakfast and lunch programs. School lunch programs started in 1946, when the Richard B. Russell National School Lunch Act, establishing the National School Lunch Program, was signed into law. The law has two purposes: (1) bolstering food prices by absorbing farm surpluses, and (2) providing low-cost or free lunches to qualifying students. Schools that participate in the program are reimbursed for meals served to qualifying students and are eligible for additional food as it becomes available from farm surpluses. About 30 million children are fed through the National School Lunch Program every school day.

The School Breakfast Program is an offshoot of the National School Lunch Program, providing subsidized breakfasts to children. As with the National School Lunch Program, schools are reimbursed for meals served to eligible children, with the degree of reimbursement depending on the economic status of the student. Schools in the program are required to offer free breakfasts to children from families with incomes below 130 percent of the federal poverty line, and children from families with incomes between 130 and 180 percent of the federal poverty line are offered breakfast at a reduced rate. Approximately 50 percent of the students fed through the National Lunch Program also participate in the School Breakfast Program, which feeds about 15 million children a day. The school breakfast and lunch programs fall under the USDA, and they are typically administered by state agencies through agreements with local school districts.

While many cities have programs providing food to low-income children and families, studies have suggested that the solution to income-based health disparity also requires increased nutritional education. Local activists and governments across the United States have developed nutrition educational programs that couple free meals with nutrition education in an effort to help people make better dietary choices. Many of these programs specifically target families that participate in the Supplemental Nutrition Assistance Program, which offers nutrition assistance to millions of low-income individuals and families.

RECOMMENDATIONS FOR CITY DWELLERS

It is impossible for individuals to guarantee the quality and availability of their food supply 100 percent of the time without having their own farm and growing their own food. However, there are steps that people can take to reduce the risk of food contamination, increase available food options, and decrease the carbon footprint of their food consumption. Some examples are listed here:

- To reduce the risk of food contamination, everyone needs to practice safe food-handling techniques, including (1) washing hands prior to handling food to avoid contamination with microorganisms and dirt; (2) washing produce before cooking or eating to rinse off any pesticides and any other harmful contaminants; (3) cooking eggs and raw meat to the appropriate temperature to kill any microorganisms; and (4) storing food appropriately to avoid spoilage and food waste.

- To reduce the amount of food that needs to be shipped to the city from rural areas, urban dwellers can grow their own fruits and vegetables. This can take many forms, from a plot in a community garden to window boxes and indoor vertical surfaces that can be used in areas with limited space.

- To reduce food waste, city residents can start a compost pile with food scraps, which will produce nutrient-rich soil that can be used for gardening. Additionally, they can consider donating some forms of unused food (e.g., unopened cans, bottles, and boxes) to food banks and other local organizations that distribute food to people in need. (It is estimated that about one in eight Americans struggles with hunger.) See Table 9 for more tips to avoid wasting food.

City residents can also get involved with food-sharing initiatives, where both food and knowledge are shared with other city residents. These initiatives take many forms, including cooking classes, food pantries, and community food kitchens. Many low-income families depend on food pantries for their daily meals, and large cities often have a sizable homeless population that sleeps in shelters or out in the open and depends on food kitchens. A good way to spend free time is to volunteer at a food pantry or kitchen, which are often sponsored by city agencies, religious organizations, and other nonprofits. Another way to volunteer is to work for Meals on Wheels, which delivers warm meals to older adults, helping them live healthier and better nourished lives in their own homes. In the United States, there are over 5,000 community-based Meals on Wheels organizations, serving virtually every large city and thousands of smaller communities.

Table 9   Additional Tips to Avoid Food Waste

Food Waste Tips	Details
Be aware of how much food you throw away.	Do not buy more food than can be used before it spoils.
Plan meals and use shopping lists.	Think about what you are buying and when it will be eaten. Check the refrigerator and pantry before going to the store to avoid buying what you already have.
Avoid impulse and bulk purchases, especially produce and dairy that have a limited shelf life.	Promotions encouraging purchases of unusual or bulk products often result in consumers buying foods outside their typical needs or family preferences, and potentially large portions of these foods may end up in the trash.
When eating out, become a more mindful eater.	If you are not terribly hungry, request smaller portions. Bring your leftovers home, refrigerate or freeze them within two hours, and check the FoodKeeper (https://www.foodsafety.gov/keep/foodkeeperapp) to see how long they will be safe to eat.
Check the temperature setting of your fridge.	Use a refrigerator thermometer to be sure that the temperature is at 40°F (4°C) or below to keep foods safe. The temperature of your freezer should be 0°F (–18°C) or below.
Avoid overpacking your refrigerator.	Cold air must circulate around refrigerated foods to keep them properly chilled.
Wipe up spills immediately.	Doing so not only reduces the growth of *Listeria* bacteria (which can grow at refrigerator temperatures), cleaning up spills (especially drips from thawing meats) also helps prevent cross-contamination, where bacteria from one food spread to another.
Keep foods covered.	Store refrigerated foods in covered containers or sealed storage bags, and check leftovers daily for spoilage.

Table 9   (continued)

Food Waste Tips	Details
Refrigerate peeled or cut vegetables.	Refrigeration is important, not only for freshness, but to keep the vegetables from going bad.
Use your freezer.	Freezing is a great way to store most foods to keep them from going bad, until you are ready to eat them. The FoodKeeper has information on how long most common foods can be stored in the freezer.
Check your fridge often.	Doing so helps keep track of what you have and what needs to be used. Eat or freeze items before you need to throw them away.
Remember the two-hour rule.	To keep foods safe when entertaining, do not leave perishable foods out for more than two hours unless you are keeping hot foods hot and cold foods cold. If you are eating outdoors and the temperature is above 90°F (32°C), perishable foods should not be left out for more than one hour.

Source: FDA.

Green Buildings and Sustainable Development

A healthy city requires healthy buildings—buildings that provide a healthy indoor environment while reducing their impact on the outside environment. Commonly called "green buildings," these are buildings that are planned, designed, constructed, and operated with serious consideration given to energy and water use, indoor environmental quality, and environmental impacts on the building site and surrounding neighborhood. They incorporate environmentally friendly mechanical systems and construction materials, use recycled materials when possible, minimize construction waste, and in busy city districts, integrate with the city's transportation infrastructure. When green buildings are part of the urban landscape, sustainable urban development is more easily attainable, and public health benefits too.

Why are buildings so important? One reason is that buildings consume huge amounts of energy. Globally, buildings account for about one-third of total energy consumption and half of electricity demand. About two-thirds of the energy that buildings consume comes from the combustion of fossil fuels—coal, oil, and natural gas—in power plants, which results in air pollution linked to urban smog and causing about 30 percent of the world's energy-related carbon dioxide (CO_2) emissions. (CO_2 is the principal global warming gas responsible for climate change.)

Another reason why buildings are important to urban health concerns the environment *inside* the building—in particular, the quality of the air that building occupants breathe. On average, adults living in developed nations spend around 90 percent of their time inside buildings—at home, work, school, stores, movie theaters, and other indoor facilities. This means that building occupants are exposed to any contaminants in the indoor air for an extended period almost every day. These contaminants can include a wide variety of gases and particulates that can cause sickness and disease, as noted in Table 10. According to the U.S. Environmental Protection Agency (EPA), "a growing body of scientific evidence has indicated that the air within homes and other buildings can be more seriously polluted than the outdoor air in even the largest and most industrialized cities." (See the "Indoor Air Quality" entry to learn more about exposures inside buildings.)

Buildings will have an even greater influence on human health and the environment in the future due to population growth and the increasing number of people moving to cities. (Already, more than half the world's population lives in urban areas.) By 2060, total building floor area (i.e., the total combined area in square feet or meters of every building in the world) is projected to double, which means that pollution from power generation will increase and many more people will be exposed to contaminants in the inside air. To put this into perspective, the existing floor area of buildings across Japan today is equal to the global floor area increase expected *every year.*

Fortunately, increases in global energy use due to new building construction will be moderated somewhat by (1) energy-efficient architectural designs for new buildings; (2) energy-saving technology retrofits for existing buildings; and (3) a greater reliance on renewable energy, such as solar and wind power. Nevertheless, building energy use throughout the world is expected to increase by roughly one-third to as much as 50 percent by the middle of the century, with nearly 80 percent of the increase occurring in developing countries and emerging economies due to population growth and greater purchasing power.

The trend toward growth in the building sector and associated energy use is concerning to city health officials tasked with addressing air pollution and climate change in the face of rising urban populations throughout much of the world. However, opportunities exist to achieve substantial energy-use reductions in buildings more quickly and at a lower cost compared with fully developing renewable energy sources, such as solar and wind power. Thus, constructing green, energy-efficient buildings and renovating existing buildings to conserve more energy are often priorities of

Table 10 Categories of Air Contaminants in Buildings That Can Cause Illnesses

Pollutant Category	Possible Sources
Biological contaminants, including mold and mildew	Bird droppings, cockroaches and rodents, condensation, cooling coils and drain pans, cooling towers, damp duct insulation or filters, damp building materials and furnishings, dust mites, humidifiers, reentrained sanitary exhausts
Chemicals in composite wood products, glues, and finishes (including formaldehyde)	Particleboard, fiberboard, plywood, other cabinetry and furniture materials, coatings, fabrics
Combustion contaminants	Furnaces, gas or kerosene space heaters, generators, tobacco products, pollutants entering the building from the outdoor air
Particles and fibers	Inside construction and renovation activities (including insulation handling), wear and tear of building materials and furnishings, paper copying and printing, building upkeep (e.g., vacuuming), occupant smoking, and pollutants entering the building from the outside air
Pesticides	Disinfectants, fungicides, herbicides, insecticides, rodenticides
Soil gases, including methane, radon, sewer gas, and volatile organic compounds	Dry drain traps, leaking underground storage tanks, nearby waste disposal sites, sewer drain leak, soil and rock (radon)
Tobacco smoke	Secondhand and thirdhand exposure to smoke from cigarettes, cigars, and pipes in the surrounding environment
Volatile organic compounds	Adhesives, air fresheners, cleansers, copy machines, dry-cleaned clothing, dyes, fuels, lubricants, paints, perfumes, pesticides, plastics, polishes, printers, sealants, solvents, stains, tobacco products, varnishes, waxes, wood preservatives

Source: EPA.

urban-sustainability programs, at least in the short term, until renewable energy is more fully established. In particular, applying technologies for reducing space-heating energy demand (accounting for over one-third of global energy use in buildings) and space cooling (the fastest-growing end-use of energy in buildings) can pay the greatest dividends in energy reductions over the shortest period. Substantial energy reductions can also be achieved with energy-efficient lighting and appliances.

In addition to energy-efficiency and indoor air quality considerations, other design features of buildings and their surroundings can help make urban areas more sustainable. These include waste management and recycling programs, pervious parking areas that allow water infiltration and reduce runoff, water-conserving fixtures and appliances, and exterior surfaces that absorb less heat than traditional building materials, helping to keep the surroundings cool. Building landscaping, including shade trees, is also important for moderating heating and cooling requirements, reducing air pollution and CO_2 concentrations, and controlling rainwater runoff, and landscaping improves mental health by creating pleasant and relaxing urban scenery. Unfortunately, as urban areas expand, the replacement of damaged and removed greenery with new landscaping is more the exception than the rule. In the United States, about 36 million trees are lost in cities every year due to urban expansion and development, where wooded and natural areas are replaced with roadways, parking lots, and other impervious surfaces.

IMPACT ON URBAN HEALTH

The electric utility power plants that provide energy to buildings in urban areas are typically located at the fringes of large metropolitan areas or in rural areas some distance from population centers. However, the air pollution from these plants can be transported through the atmosphere over long distances, contributing to city ozone and particulate pollution and affecting the health of urban residents. Additionally, large manufacturing facilities with their own electric power generation capabilities can contribute to urban air pollution. People who are more sensitive to air pollution—children, older adults, pregnant women, and people with preexisting health conditions—are often the first to suffer the effects of ozone and particulates. Additionally, some low-income and minority communities that are located close to freeways and industrial facilities are at greater risk of compromised health because they are exposed to higher levels of air pollution than are residents who live in less polluted suburban neighborhoods and can afford better healthcare. The mix of air pollutants found in polluted urban areas is associated with:

- asthma attacks and shortness of breath
- harmful respiratory and cardiovascular system effects
- aggravated lung diseases
- permanent damage to lungs through long-term exposure
- increased hospitalizations and emergency room visits for heart attacks and strokes
- premature death

When urban air pollution episodes combine with summer heat waves, the outcome can be deadly, particularly for older residents and others with pre-existing health conditions.

Health issues are a concern inside buildings too. It is somewhat common for building occupants to complain about odors, stale and stuffy air, and symptoms of illness, and these complaints may have worsened in recent years, as building have become better insulated and more airtight to reduce heating and air-conditioning losses. In many cases, the discomfort experienced inside some buildings is caused by conditions such as poor temperature regulation and low humidity, which can be remedied through heating and air-conditioning adjustments, air humidification, and ventilation improvements. However, in other cases, occupants have become seriously ill due to contaminants in the building where they live or work, raising serious concerns about building design and maintenance. The causes of indoor discomfort and diseases are often very difficult to diagnose, although poor ventilation is believed to be implicated (i.e., causing or worsening the problem) in about half of the cases.

Inside exposure to contaminants is often categorized as either acute or chronic, which are defined as follows:

- **Acute exposure**. Acute health problems generally occur within 24 hours following exposure, and these effects generally (but not always) disappear soon after exposure ends. Two examples are (1) certain volatile organic chemicals released from building materials that cause headaches and (2) mold spores released from damp materials or air-handling systems that can sometimes cause itchy eyes and runny noses. Occasionally, short-term exposure to certain biocontaminants, such as fungi, bacteria, and viruses, can cause serious, long-lasting respiratory diseases.

- **Chronic exposure.** The health problems associated with chronic or repeated exposures can be quite serious and sometimes debilitating, even at low exposure levels. Some substances in the indoor air, such as asbestos, benzene, radon, and environmental tobacco smoke, may even increase the risk of developing cancer.

Building occupants may also suffer from excessive or too little light, blue light from computers, excessive noise, and lead in drinking water (a growing concern in U.S. schools). In addition to making building occupants sick, uncomfortable indoor conditions can affect employee performance by reducing the ability of workers to concentrate and perform basic mental and physical tasks. Occasionally, building occupants are afflicted with sick building syndrome and Legionnaires' disease (potentially serious health conditions described in the "Indoor Air Quality" entry).

Buildings can also affect urban health in more indirect ways, such as by enhancing the heat island effect. The buildings and roadways in cities are made of a variety of dense construction materials—concrete, asphalt, stone, brick, and steel. These dense materials absorb energy from the sun, leading to warmer days, as well as to warmer evenings as these materials release their heat to the surrounding air. This is called the "heat island effect," and it can cause city temperatures during daylight hours to be up to 5°F (2.8°C) higher than surrounding areas for a typical city with a population of 1 million or more. The effect is more pronounced at night, when city temperatures can be up to 22°F (12.2°C) higher than surrounding areas. This excess heat can lead to more energy consumption for air conditioning, higher air pollution levels, and more heat-related discomfort and illness, such as respiratory difficulties, heat cramps and exhaustion, and heat stroke. Because trees can have a moderating effect on surrounding temperatures, cutting down trees to make room for new building construction can exacerbate the heat island effect.

WHAT CITIES ARE DOING ABOUT BUILDING DESIGN AND SUSTAINABLE DEVELOPMENT

Most major cities throughout the world have building codes aimed at ensuring safe construction practices and building integrity, and it is becoming more common for these codes to also include requirements for energy efficiency and the use of renewable power. Such requirements, which may be mandatory or voluntary, are especially important in developing countries, where rapid urbanization and economic development are causing a boom in building construction. Building codes are usually applied to new construction, but some existing buildings are also subject to codes (e.g., during certain maintenance activities, renovations, and expansions). Building codes can be prescriptive, although the international trend is more toward performance-based codes or a combination of prescriptive and performance-based codes. Prescriptive-based codes require specific design elements and materials, whereas performance-based codes require a specified energy performance to be demonstrated, usually through modeling assessments during the design stage and sometimes verified during building operations.

In the United States, codes in California are by far the most progressive, where several cities require new homes to include solar power or other clean-energy sources, and the state will require all new homes to have solar power beginning in 2020. (This requirement will apply to single-family homes and to multifamily buildings up to three stories high, and homes often shaded from the sun are exempt.) The price tag for residential solar installations in California is estimated to range from $8,000 to $12,000 on average, which will add around $40 to the typical 30-year monthly mortgage payment. These costs are expected to be more than offset by the savings in heating, cooling, and lighting costs, which for the typical home will be around $80 per month. Already, solar energy provides about 16 percent of California's electricity, and over 80,000 workers are employed in the solar industry.

In addition to codes, various types of incentives are often available from city, state, and federal governments to encourage energy efficiency in building design and operation. These include

- tax credits, deductions, and exemptions
- equipment rebates and discounts
- loans, grants, and financing programs
- weatherization assistance
- energy-efficient mortgages (mortgages that provide more borrowing power by giving credit for a home's energy efficiency)
- net-metering and feed-in tariffs (programs that encourage investment in renewable energy by allowing homeowners and other power-company customers to feed energy back into the electric grid)

An excellent compilation of U.S. clean energy policies and incentives is available online through the Database of State Incentives for Renewables and Efficiency (dsireusa.org).

Globally, the United Nations Development Programme encourages market demand for public and private investment in energy efficiency through a variety of policy, financial, and assistance programs aimed at households, public and municipal facilities, and residential and commercial buildings. Also, it helps local and national governments design and adopt efficient policies and legislation. Many other organizations throughout the world also promote energy-efficient buildings as essential building blocks of a sustainable urban environment.

Building energy certifications have become very popular in recent years as buyers and occupants are attracted to the environmental-sustainability features of energy-efficient buildings, as well as to their lower operating costs. These certifications are similar to codes, in that certain energy standards must be achieved, although certification programs tend to be more prescriptive, sometimes covering building materials, water use, and waste generation and extending beyond the building envelope to features such as landscaping, water drainage, impervious parking surfaces, and onsite renewable energy systems. In addition to having lower energy costs, certified buildings help reduce greenhouse gas (GHG) emissions and other air pollutants, resulting in significant benefits to public health in urban areas while contributing to the fight against climate change. Certified buildings also often provide healthy indoor environments to live, work, and play in. Nearly 40 countries have mandatory certification programs in place or under development, and voluntary programs have been established in 80 countries.

One popular building-certification program based in the United States is Leadership in Energy and Environmental Design (LEED), sponsored by the U.S. Green Building Council. LEED, claiming to be the most widely used green building rating system in the world, certifies virtually all building types, including major renovations, and it has a presence in over 165 countries and territories. A related program called LEED for Cities is designed to help urban areas become more sustainable by allowing cities to measure and manage citywide water consumption, energy use, waste generation, transportation, and the overall human experience. Another LEED program, LEED Neighborhood, is designed to help create more sustainable neighborhoods, looking beyond the scale of buildings to the entire community.

City codes, initiatives, and certifications have made great strides over the past 25 years in creating healthy and sustainable buildings and communities. However, about two-thirds of global building energy use is still not subject to energy-performance standards, and much more progress is needed if the world is to avoid the severe consequences of climate change. The Global Alliance for Buildings and Construction (GABC), an international alliance of national and local authorities, international organizations, companies, civil societies, and financial institutions, has identified the following urgent priorities for the building and construction sector:

- **Urban-planning policies for energy efficiency**—use urban-planning policies to affect the form and compactness of buildings to enable reduced energy demand and increased renewable-energy capacity.

- **Improve the performance of existing buildings**—increase the energy-efficiency-renovation rate and increase the level of energy efficiency in existing buildings.

- **Achieve net-zero operating emissions**—increase the uptake of building- or system-level net-zero operating emissions for new buildings.

- **Improve energy management of all buildings**—reduce the operating energy and emissions through improved energy management tools and operational capacity building.

- **Decarbonize energy**—integrate renewable energy and reduce the carbon footprint of energy demand in buildings.

- **Reduce embodied energy and emissions**—reduce the environmental impact of materials and equipment in buildings and the construction value chain by taking a life-cycle approach.

- **Reduce energy demand from appliances**—collaborate with global initiatives to reduce the energy demand from appliances, lighting, and cooking.

- **Upgrade adaptation**—reduce climate change–related risks of buildings by adapting building design and improving resilience.

- **Increase awareness**—support training and capacity building, including educational and informative tools to make the case for sustainable buildings and construction.

Perhaps the most important—and most challenging—of these goals is to achieve net-zero operating emissions, which means to eliminate net GHG emissions from the homes, offices, shops, stadiums, theaters, and industrial buildings of the future by powering these facilities with renewable energy, such as solar and wind power. (More rigorously, the net-zero concept can be applied to a building's entire life cycle, from raw material extraction to the building's ultimate deconstruction and disposal many years into the future.) According to the GABC, "there is a critical window of opportunity to address buildings and construction in the coming decade to avoid lock-in of inefficient buildings over the next 40 years [and] to address energy performance improvements and emissions reduction in the world's existing buildings stock. Swift and ambitious action is needed without delay to avoid locking in inefficient buildings assets for decades to come."

To provide a safe and healthy indoor environment for residents, many cities address indoor air quality through zoning laws, construction permits, and local ordinances. For example, landlords may be required to keep buildings clean, sanitary, and pest-free, and building contractors may need to meet the latest best practices for heating, air conditioning, ventilation, building materials, and smoke and carbon monoxide alarms. Also, many cities prohibit smoking in public spaces and specify procedures for renovating or demolishing old buildings containing lead paint or asbestos insulation.

RECOMMENDATIONS FOR CITY DWELLERS

There are a number of actions that urban dwellers can take at home to avoid wasting energy while improving the indoor environment. Furthermore, commercial and industrial building managers may be receptive to ideas for reducing energy use (which cuts operating costs) and improving the indoor environment (which reduces occupant complaints and potential litigation). By helping to conserve energy and reduce energy losses at home and where they work and shop, city residents can fight climate change and improve the urban environment by reducing GHGs and other air pollutants from power plants that burn fossil fuels.

Actions to reduce building energy loss include (1) carefully insulating and sealing walls, ceilings, and floors; (2) installing high-quality insulated windows; (3) purchasing energy-efficient appliances (e.g., appliances carrying the *Energy Star* label); (4) installing renewable-energy technology, such as solar panels, wind power, and solar hot water heaters; (5) constructing or purchasing buildings with windows oriented to capture the winter sunlight and shaded to prevent overheating in the summer months; and (6) incorporating solar mass (i.e., dense building materials that help reduce wintertime heating costs by absorbing heat from sunlight during daylight hours and slowly releasing it in the evening). Modifying occupant behavior can also be effective at reducing building energy use. For example, teaching homeowners to turn the thermostat back 10°F–15°F (5.6°C–8.3°C) while sleeping at night or when away from home can reduce heating and cooling bills by about 10 percent per year. Many utility companies offer incentives or rebates to encourage the installation of energy-efficient lighting and appliances, and a number of excellent books are available on how to design and live in energy-efficient buildings.

When modern buildings are highly insulated and well sealed to prevent energy loss, indoor air-quality problems sometimes can occur because the exchange between indoor and outside air is reduced. (Providing adequate air exchange is not as great a problem with many older buildings, where air flows more freely through cracks in the walls, floors, and ceilings and around windows, although these buildings also may experience infiltration of air pollution from the outside air.) Solutions to the buildup of air contaminants in tightly sealed modern buildings include installing ventilation systems that conserve energy (sometimes called "heat recovery ventilators" or "energy recovery ventilators") and furnaces that carefully regulate intake air to provide just the right number of air exchanges per hour. These techniques provide adequate ventilation while reducing heat or air conditioning losses. Buildings that incorporate balanced ventilation fans for both inlet and exhaust airflow, or that facilitate natural ventilation through design considerations, can also be effective, particularly during seasons when heat or air conditioning losses are not a concern. Consult with a building contractor or manager to investigate these and other techniques for ensuring clean indoor air for you, your family, and your coworkers.

CITY SPOTLIGHT: SINGAPORE—PROVING DENSELY POPULATED CITIES CAN BE BOTH LIVABLE AND SUSTAINABLE

Cities with high population densities can suffer from congested roadways, crowded markets, long commutes to work and school, and in some parts of the world, poverty and disease. In contrast, densely populated Singapore has found a way to create a healthy and vibrant cityscape amid a multitude of high-rises and explosive economic growth.

What Singapore has accomplished since gaining independence in 1965 is truly astounding. Once characterized by slums, open sewers, and poverty, with limited land area and no natural resources to speak of, the future of this city-state, island nation looked bleak. Today, however, Singapore is a thriving global financial center and the envy of the world for its rapid economic growth and high standard of living for its nearly 6 million inhabitants. It is an unlikely candidate for high livability given its extreme population density, which at over 20,000 people per square mile (8,000 people per square kilometer) ranks third among nations.

Surrounded by water, outward expansion is not an option for Singapore. Thus, as the city-state develops, it has little choice but to expand vertically through the construction of a multitude of high-rise buildings, many providing housing for its residents. To guide this construction, visionary city planners created the concept of "livable density," which means putting people first in designing urban developments. Through innovative planning, building codes, and zoning, the city-state has become a highly livable locale, where most residents enjoy good health, a pleasant and clean environment, and plenty of amenities.

The city-state accomplished this through an integrated approach involving sustainable building standards, mixed-use development zoning, and requirements for buildings to incorporate greenery, such as green roofs, vertical gardens, and green walls. Parks, streams, and ponds are interspersed among the high-rise buildings, providing respite from the surrounding steel, glass, and concrete, and greenery is visible just about everywhere you look. There is even a stand of virgin rainforest preserved in the center of the island. With all the streetside plantings, parks and gardens between tall buildings, and green roofs, the view from above reveals a lush canopy of green foliage covering almost half of the city-state.

Singapore's high-rise neighborhoods are carefully designed to ensure that residents have ready access to work, school, shopping, entertainment, and healthcare facilities, usually within a short walk. Also, public transportation is among the best in the world, and Singapore's parks, while limited compared with other large urban areas, are connected with a network of paths, making walking or bicycling around the city-state easy. Through innovative urban planning and high-rise architectural design, an illusion of space is created that is missing from other densely populated urban areas, such as Manhattan in New York City or downtown London. The city-state's ability to achieve harmony among so many diverse urban elements is truly unique.

One guiding principle of Singapore's development is to embrace its cultural diversity. With many Chinese, Indians, Malaysians, and other ethnicities living in such close proximity, city planners recognized the importance making everyone feel included in the social fabric. Thus, Singapore encourages cultural events and celebrates its many traditions and cuisines.

Another unique feature of Singapore's urban planning is a commitment to finding a way for almost everyone to be a homeowner. In doing so, residents become more invested in the future of the city-state and have more financial security. Housing apartments built by the government housing and development board are made affordable with 99-year financing, and prices are set so that a family spends no more than a quarter of its income on housing. Today, there are almost 1 million apartment units housing over 80 percent of the population, and virtually all are privately owned by the residents. Older adult owners can sublet their units or sell part of their ownership back to the city-state, using the proceeds for a retirement annuity.

Successful high-density, high-rise urban developments like Singapore's are not without criticism. In Singapore, critics point out that many children exhibit symptoms of depression, perhaps because the city's commerce-oriented maze of high-rises, along with subway stations, office complexes, and underground shopping malls, are not particularly conducive to spontaneous play and exploration of the natural environment. And childhood development experts contend that high-rise housing, no matter how well designed and luxurious, can never provide a favorable setting for raising children. Research shows that young adults in Singapore are becoming less interested in dating—a perplexing phenomenon that may suggest stress or reduced self-esteem among young people.

Critics also note that modern high-rises can be sterile, isolating, and stifling to creativity, whereas creativity seems to thrive in urban environments like San Francisco's Mission District or London's East End, with their stimulating mix of coffee shops, specialty stores, restaurants, and perhaps an old warehouse turned into an art gallery or condominium. Schools in Singapore are addressing these concerns by providing more creative experiences in the classroom. Also, city planners believe mixed-use developments can be very stimulating with the right design.

Singapore's successful experience as a high-density urban environment illustrates how other densely populated cities can also achieve a high quality of life through innovative mixed-use architectural designs, affordable home ownership, extensive greenery, and a commitment to putting people first in the urban-planning process. Furthermore, cityscapes like Singapore's can become more resilient and sustainable through modern public transportation systems, green building codes, and easily accessible walkways and bicycle paths. Also, urban areas that are similar to Singapore, with many trees and gardens, tend to be cooler and less troubled by air pollution.

Green Space and Natural Areas

"Green space" is any piece of land in a city that is undeveloped and covered with grass, trees, shrubs, or other vegetation. Examples are parks, community gardens, schoolyards, cemeteries, vacant lots, and public plazas planted with greenery. Additionally, a green roof, which is a rooftop covered with vegetation, might also be considered green space. "Natural areas" are parts of a city that are largely undisturbed from their natural state, such as wooded areas, meadows, and wetlands. Green spaces and natural areas are important for recreation, relaxation, health, and the environment, and they add to the aesthetic appeal of a neighborhood.

Green spaces and natural areas are fundamental components of the "urban ecosystem," which is the complex community of humans, animals, and plants living among the buildings and roadways of a city. For a city to provide a healthy environment for its citizens, its urban ecosystem must support the services and opportunities that a society needs to prosper and be happy. Green spaces and natural areas help create a healthy urban ecosystem by:

- providing areas for relaxation and recreation in a pleasant setting
- creating a refuge from the noise and commotion of the city
- moderating temperatures and countering the urban heat island effect
- helping fight climate change by removing carbon dioxide (CO_2) from the surrounding air
- reducing air pollution by filtering gases and particles

- capturing rainwater, thereby helping to recharge aquifers and prevent urban flooding
- encouraging physical activity, such as walking, jogging, and bicycling
- facilitating social interactions in beautiful surroundings

It is no coincidence that many great thinkers have taken walks through city parks for inspiration, or as Henry David Thoreau (1817–1862) put it, "Methinks that the moment my legs begin to move, my thoughts begin to flow." American science journalist Ferris Jabr explains it this way: "Because we don't have to devote much conscious effort to the act of walking, our attention is free to wander—to overlay the world before us with a parade of images from the mind's theatre. This is precisely the kind of mental state that studies have linked to innovative ideas and strokes of insight." Just about every health expert agrees that time spent in an urban green space or natural area, whether walking, exercising, or simply stretching out in the grass, is time well spent for one's mental health.

One type of green space is a "green street," which is an approach to stormwater management that incorporates vegetation (e.g., trees and shrubs), soil, and permeable pavement for the purpose of slowing, filtering, and cleansing stormwater runoff from streets, parking areas, and sidewalks. Green streets capture rainwater where it falls, rather than allowing it to drain into storm sewers or directly into surface waters that serve as the public water supply. This helps prevent up to 90 percent of roadway and landscaping contaminants from entering nearby bodies of water while keeping sewers from backing up in heavy rains, and by capturing rainfall on permeable surfaces, green streets help recharge groundwater aquifers. In addition to their stormwater management features, green streets may incorporate park benches, energy-efficient lighting, bicycle lanes, and other elements that help create a pleasant, almost parklike environment for shopping and conducting other business in a city. Green streets facilitate healthy activities like walking and bicycling, and the greenery helps keep the city cooler on hot summer days.

A concept related to green streets is "green infrastructure," which uses a variety of green spaces, such as parks, lawns, gardens, wooded areas, and streets lined with trees and planters, to capture rainfall, prevent urban flooding, and generally create a healthier urban environment. Additionally, green infrastructure helps reduce air and water pollution, improve groundwater quantity and quality, and provide habitat for urban wildlife. One type of green infrastructure, a "rain garden," is a shallow, vegetated basin that collects and absorbs rainwater runoff from roofs and paved areas. Rain gardens mimic the processes of infiltration, evaporation, and transpiration that take place in natural areas, and they also help make the urban landscape more attractive. "Planter boxes" are rain gardens on a small scale that are ideal for busy urban streets and restricted areas, and "bioswales" are rain gardens placed in the long, narrow spaces between sidewalks and curbs. Another type of green infrastructure is a "rainwater harvesting system," which collects rainwater from building roofs and other architectural features, channeling it into rain barrels or other collection systems for later use (e.g., landscape irrigation).

Green spaces and natural areas are an integral part of the concept known as "smart growth," which is a strategy designed to protect public health and the environment in urban areas while helping make communities more attractive, economically stronger, and socially diverse. As vacant urban areas undergo development, and as blighted areas are redeveloped, many cities employ a number of smart-growth approaches, depending on local circumstances. For example, when neighborhoods are designed to include parks, homes, offices, schools, and houses of worship in the same general area, residents walk, ride bicycles, and enjoy the outdoors more often, and the physical and emotional stress that often comes with busy city life is reduced. Also, there is less pollution, and natural areas in the surroundings are often preserved. Smart-growth policies often result in attractive, aesthetically pleasing communities that foster a strong sense of place among the inhabitants.

IMPACT ON URBAN HEALTH

Urban dwellers are naturally attracted to parks and other green spaces, and it is not surprising that the highest property values in a city are often in areas adjoining a city park. The time people spend in green spaces—walking a dog, playing games, or having a picnic—benefits both physical and mental health by providing physical exercise and relieving mental stress. Green spaces are also conducive to spontaneous social interactions as people strike up conversations with friends and neighbors they encounter while strolling in parks and along green streets.

Research into the time that people spend in green spaces and natural areas has uncovered a range of lasting health benefits, including lower blood pressure and reduced cholesterol levels, more rapid recovery from surgery, longer survival after a heart attack, less self-reported stress, and fewer medical complaints overall. Studies also show that children and teens with attention and behavioral disorders can experience significant improvements when spending more time in contact with nature. Other research suggests that exercise is more beneficial when it occurs in natural settings instead of along busy urban streets.

Another advantage of urban green spaces and natural areas is that they help increase overall fitness and reduce obesity for people willing to take advantage of these amenities. Being fit can help with obesity-related conditions like diabetes, and some studies have shown that physically active individuals have lower medical costs. Also, older adults who are active park users were observed to have fewer trips to the doctor's office, and their level of physical activity was found to be the strongest predictor of lower blood pressure. Factors that contribute to the level of activity in parks and other green spaces include proximity and ease of accessibility, good lighting for nighttime activities, readily accessible toilets and water fountains, well-designed and -maintained paths, and attractive scenery. An interesting study performed in Tokyo, the world's largest metropolitan area, found that for retired people on pensions, living near parks and tree-lined streets had the greatest impact on lifespan, even when accounting for other factors that affect longevity, including gender, marital status, income, and age.

An added benefit of green spaces and natural areas to public health is that they help reduce air and water pollution, climate change, and urban heating. These benefits occur because green areas (1) absorb air pollutants, including the primary greenhouse gas (GHG), CO_2; (2) cleanse rainwater and stormwater runoff as water filters through soil and recharges groundwater aquifers; and (3) cool the surrounding air by providing shade and by reducing the quantity of dense materials in the city, like concrete and asphalt, that absorb heat from the sun. Also, cooling is achieved by the process of "transpiration," where moisture evaporates from the leaves on trees and other foliage using energy in the form of heat taken from the surrounding air. Parks and natural areas within cities can be as much as 5°F–10°F (3°C–6°C) cooler than other urban areas due to the effects of transpiration and shading. Because cities cooled by extensive greenery require less energy to power air conditioners, there is less energy-associated pollution, such as the toxic air contaminants emitted from fossil fuel–burning power plants.

Green areas within a city also benefit health by providing opportunities for social connection and networking. People are more inclined to engage in conversation, even with strangers, as they relax in a natural setting, and researchers have discovered that these social connections are valuable in reducing stress and providing a sense of connection with the community. This is especially important for older adults, who often experience social isolation while living in the city. The networking that occurs in parks and along green streets helps people get to know each other better, learn about city resources and services, and establish a web of friends to call upon in times of need. In short, the relationships that develop through social interactions in city parks and other green areas are crucial to the social fabric of a city.

Finally, the importance of urban gardens (also called "community gardens") to public health cannot be overstated. Many urban dwellers, especially in larger cities, live in "food deserts," which are areas largely void of fresh fruits, vegetables, and other healthful unprocessed foods. This is especially an issue in impoverished areas inhabited by low-income people, who may not be able to afford fresh foods even if they were available locally. Urban gardens are helping to address this problem by providing local access to affordable fresh foods, frequently at minimal or no cost. These gardens are generally collaborative projects organized by local citizens, where participants share in gardening activities and receive produce in return, and cities often support these endeavors by donating vacant lots or portions of public lands for the garden plots. (Sometimes some of the best gardeners are immigrants who tended farms or gardens in their home countries before moving to the United States.) In addition to providing healthy foods, urban gardens help people be physically active and strengthen social connections, all while creating pleasing green areas within the city.

WHAT CITIES ARE DOING ABOUT GREEN SPACE AND NATURAL AREAS

Most city managers these days recognize the importance of green space and natural areas for public health, as well as tourism and commercial development, and city development plans routinely include parks, green streets, urban gardens, and other green areas. Because people of different ages, socioeconomic groups, and cultural backgrounds may have different habits, traditions, and attitudes when it come to physical activity and exercise, cities typically incorporate a variety of green areas in diverse configurations and locations, including lower-income areas for city residents who are economically disadvantaged and lack access to a gym or other exercise facility.

Some urban green areas are small, squeezed into alleys between high-rise buildings in busy commercial districts, while other areas are as expansive as Central Park in New York City. And while some green areas take the form of traditional parks, others are more innovative, like the High Line, a popular New York public park built on a historic freight rail line elevated above the streets on Manhattan's West Side. (The High Line includes perennials, grasses, shrubs, and trees displaying a variety of textures and colors in all four seasons.) Atlanta similarly transformed an old railroad corridor, this time at ground level, into a greenway encircling the downtown area, connecting 45 neighborhoods and a number of parks.

Many other cities have also discovered innovative ways to incorporate green areas into the urban landscape. For example, in Dallas, Klyde Warren Park comprises a 5-acre (2-hectare) deck constructed over the top of an eight-lane highway, creating a pleasant, parklike environment that allows pedestrians and bicyclists to travel between the uptown area and the Dallas arts district. Millennium Park in Chicago, once an industrial wasteland, now includes a 5-acre (2-hectare) perennial garden and world-class concert venue designed by the famous architect Frank Gehry. By sitting above a parking garage, the 24.5-acre (9.9-hectare) Millennium Park is one of the largest green roofs in the world. In Birmingham, Alabama, Railroad Park's 19 acres (7.7 hectares) of green space includes many water features, trails for walking and jogging, a biofiltration wetlands area, breathtaking views of the city, and the Birmingham History Wall. Many objects from the undeveloped railroad site, such as hand-cast bricks and original cobblestones, are used throughout the Birmingham park. Located in the shadow of Tennessee's State Capitol Building, Nashville's Bicentennial Capital Mall—named one of the top 10 public spaces in the United States—includes a 19-acre (7.7-hectare) park, a state history museum, a 200-foot (61-meter) granite map of the state, a World War II memorial, and a 95-bell carillon. A total of 11 planters along the mall's Walkway of Counties contain native species from different regions of the state.

In addition to green spaces and natural areas like those illustrated here, other green elements typically incorporated into the urban landscape include permeable pavement, rain gardens and urban gardens, and bioswales in roadway medians and along roads and parking areas. Many cities have established tree-canopy goals to help restore trees lost to development, and some cities encourage new building construction to include vegetation on rooftops to help cool the city while creating an alternative type of green space for people to enjoy. (Green roofs also filter stormwater while helping building managers reduce energy costs for cooling.) Many cities are purchasing natural areas and other open spaces within the watersheds that feed their urban water resources, with the goal of protecting these sensitive areas from development and preventing contamination of the water supply. These areas also help absorb and cleanse stormwater runoff from nearby roadways and parking lots, and by leaving the areas undisturbed, erosion of nearby streams can be avoided

Paris is another city to discover an innovative way to create green space. When looking for opportunities to address the devastating series of heat waves that have recently afflicted the city, investigations revealed that Paris has more than 750 impermeable, asphalt-covered schoolyards that contribute significantly to urban warming by absorbing heat from the sun. Paris's Schoolyard Oasis project aims to replace all this asphalt with porous materials, vegetation, water features (e.g., fountains and water sprayers), and shaded structures, thereby transforming the schoolyards into "urban cooling islands." An added value to this approach is that the city creates more green space and recreational areas, while capturing and filtering stormwater. Most important, the Schoolyard Oasis project will enhance the lives of school-age children by creating an environment more conducive to learning and sports. The average Parisian lives within just 650 feet (200 meters) of a schoolyard, and eventually, these green spaces may be opened to local residents for recreation after school hours and to older adults during heat waves.

RECOMMENDATIONS FOR CITY DWELLERS

The busy life that many city dwellers experience makes it hard to enjoy the outdoors, a critical ingredient to healthy living and good mental health. Professional jobs in the city often involve long hours, and people in the service industry frequently work two or three jobs just to make ends meet. Who has time to exercise? But when parks and other green areas are nearby, it is easier to be motivated to exercise or just sit and enjoy a peaceful moment away from the city's noise and traffic congestion. If your neighborhood does not include any green areas, consider working with a local community organization to create an urban garden or convert a vacant lot into a small park. Also, there may public green spaces nearby that you may not have thought about visiting, for example, a public plaza planted with trees, a schoolyard open to the public after school hours, or a cemetery that allows walking or viewing their flower gardens.

Remember that some form of regular exercise is necessary to stay healthy. For overall cardiovascular health, the American Heart Association recommends at least 150 minutes per week of moderate exercise or 75 minutes per week of vigorous exercise (or a combination of moderate and vigorous activity). For people who enjoy walking, an easy way to be sure to get the right amount of exercise is to walk 30 minutes per day, 5 days per week. Even if this time is divided into 10- or 15-minute segments throughout the week, healthy benefits will accrue. And if more vigorous exercise is preferred, several runs through the park or workouts at a local gym every week can help improve and maintain health.

Exercise in parks or other green areas can help you feel better about yourself too. According to the Mayo Clinic, "the links between depression, anxiety, and exercise aren't entirely clear—but working out and other forms of physical activity can definitely ease symptoms of depression or anxiety and make you feel better." Of course, check with your doctor before starting a new exercise program to make sure that it is safe for you, and if depression or anxiety symptoms interfere with your daily activities, see your doctor or mental health professional right away.

CITY SPOTLIGHT: MELBOURNE—THE MANY BENEFITS OF MORE TREES

Faced with rapidly rising temperatures and heat waves, officials in Melbourne were pressed to find a solution. Their approach—creating an urban forest—not only cools the city, but helps fight climate change and gives residents more access to nature.

Like many cities throughout the world, Melbourne, Australia, is warming up. Daytime temperatures in Melbourne recently have been dangerously hot, not only threatening human health, but contributing to raging bush fires on the edge of town and melting asphalt on a highway leading into the city. Using sophisticated climate models, researchers at the Australian National University have calculated that by 2040, summer heat waves in Melbourne could reach 122°F (50°C), even if the nations signing on to the 2015 Paris climate agreement fully meet their commitments.

Given the near-inevitability of continued warming, Melbourne officials have embarked on a major initiative to increase the number of trees in the city—planting 3,000 trees every year while protecting the health of the city's existing tree stock. Trees help keep the city cool by providing shade and reflecting heat away from streets and sidewalks. Additionally, trees provide cooling through the process of transpiration, where the evaporation of water from leaves takes heat from the surrounding air, thereby having a cooling effect.

Cooling the city with trees benefits public health in Melbourne by reducing the frequency and severity of heat waves, removing air pollutants, filtering rainwater, and providing shade from sunlight exposure. Furthermore, parks and other areas planted with trees create pleasant settings for relaxation and recreational activities, which benefits both physical and mental health. Urban green spaces are particularly therapeutic for children by encouraging creativity, exploration, and adventure and by promoting physical activity. Trees remove the primary global warming gas, CO_2, from the air, thereby helping Melbourne contribute to the goals of the 2015 Paris climate agreement.

Planting lots of trees is part of Melbourne's broader strategy to develop an urban forest, although this is not a forest in the traditional sense. Instead, an urban forest comprises all of the trees and other vegetation scattered throughout the city (e.g., in parks, gardens, plazas, campuses, and building landscapes). Also, urban forests include greenery along streets and on green roofs—rooftops planted with vegetation that helps keep buildings cooler. Many people are surprised to learn that urban forests can support a wide ranges of species by contributing to biodiversity and habitat protection, and in some urban areas, urban forests even help protect endangered species and other animals with a high conservation value.

While developing an urban forest sounds like a great idea, implementing the concept in Melbourne faces a major problem: An irreversible decline is occurring in the city's existing tree population, caused by a decade of drought and water restrictions and worsened by the presence of many trees weakened by old age. If no action is taken, the city could lose 40 percent or more of its existing tree population in the next two decades. Thus, the challenge to Melbourne in creating an expansive urban forest is not just planting new trees, but keeping the current stock of trees healthy. Another challenge is managing future urban growth, which threatens to replace stands of trees with commercial developments and roadways.

To address these concerns, the city has created a detailed urban forest strategy aimed at increasing the canopy cover (the amount of surface area covered by trees and other vegetation) to 40 percent by 2040, and achieving greater tree diversity by limiting the urban forest to no more than 5 percent of any tree species, 10 percent of any genus, and 20 percent of any one family. (The city's tree population, currently dominated by just three species, is vulnerable if one or two of the species succumbs to disease or heat stress.) Additionally, Melbourne has plans for improving overall vegetation health, increasing soil moisture and water quality, enriching the urban ecology, and enhancing the biodiversity that contributes to a healthy ecosystem. Another strategic goal is to engage residents, business leaders, and educational institutions in supporting the urban forest concept and to assist local groups working for more greenery in neighborhoods.

Melbourne's urban forest strategy runs through 2032, with the goal of achieving a significant cooling of the city as the climate becomes increasingly warm, dry, and subject to more frequent extremes of heat and inundation. If it can overcome all the obstacles and make continuous progress toward this goal, it will be well on its way to creating a healthy, livable city while helping to achieve international targets for reducing GHGs. Additionally, a greener city will result in reduced energy expenditures, increased property values, and more tourism dollars, and gains will be seen in the pedestrian economy as cooler sidewalks and streets attract more shoppers.

Healthcare Access and Quality

At least 10 percent of the U.S. population does not have access to basic healthcare services, including primary care and prevention; and worldwide, the figure is closer to 50 percent. Physician shortages and the high cost of healthcare prevent many people from getting the medical attention they need, and as a result, injuries and illnesses often go untreated. This global crisis in healthcare access and quality is particularly a problem in urban areas, where residents may be exposed to multiple health risks, and where inner-city poverty may preclude even the most basic healthcare services for a large segment of the population. Inadequate healthcare accounts for about 10 percent of premature mortality worldwide.

Although cities generally offer the best healthcare services and the widest range of specialized care, there is a chronic shortage of urban primary-care providers, even in developed nations like the United States. In many of the poorest U.S. neighborhoods, hospitals are closing and primary-care physicians are relocating to more affluent municipalities, creating urban shortage areas (i.e., fewer than one physician per 3,500 people). According to a 2018 report by the Association of Medical Colleges, the United States could see a shortage of up to 120,000 physicians by 2030, due in part to population growth and the increased medical needs of the aging U.S. population. The number of Americans over age 65 will increase by 50 percent by 2030, including many active physicians who may decide to retire, making the doctor shortage even worse.

According to a 2017 health indicators report by the Organisation for Economic Cooperation and Development (OECD), U.S. healthcare spending, at about $10,000 per person, is much higher than the other 35 OECD member-states (averaging about $4,000 per person). Even so, according to the OECD, "High cost of health care is a barrier to access for many Americans, with important shares of the population uninsured or underinsured. Indeed, 22% of the population skipped consultations and 18% did not purchase prescribed medicines due to cost in 2016. The access problem is particularly marked for poorer families, with 43% of low-income adults reporting unmet care needs because of the cost of care." Another problem in the United States is that some urban immigrant families do not seek out healthcare services because they are afraid of being deported, even if their children are American citizens.

While the United States ranks high in healthcare spending, it is below the OECD median value for life expectancy, as illustrated in Table 11. This is a complex problem involving many factors, including healthcare costs, access to health insurance, diet and lifestyle, and cultural and sociological influences. One risk factor that particularly stands out for the United States is the prevalence of obesity which, at 38 percent of adults, is well above the OECD average of about 20 percent. Furthermore, 70 percent of Americans are considered either overweight or obese, conditions associated with many health problems, including type 2 diabetes, high blood pressure, joint problems, and gallstones. Whether one is classified as overweight or obese is determined by the body mass index (BMI), a measure of body fat based on height and weight. Another worrying characteristic of U.S. healthcare concerns the number of doctors per person, which, at 2.6 per 1,000 people, is below the OECD average of 3.4. Similarly, the number of U.S. hospital beds, at 2.8 beds per 1,000 people, is below the OECD average of 4.7. On the positive side, the United States does better than the OECD average in having a low smoking rate and reduced levels of air pollution.

While issues in healthcare delivery remain to be solved in many OECD countries, including the United States, healthcare access and quality are far worse in many non-OECD countries, where hospitals and clinics are often inadequately funded and doctors are in short supply, particularly those practicing in specialty areas. Another problem in many of these countries is that health outcomes are strongly tied to socioeconomic status (an index of education, income, and occupation). This is especially true among the world's 800 million slum dwellers, representing about one-third of the global urban population. In some developing cities, where the slum population can reach up to 80 percent, healthcare is marginal or nonexistent. Many of the poorest residents see a doctor only when their health condition becomes

Table 11 Life Expectancy at Birth of Selected Countries

Country	Life Expectancy (years)
Japan	84.1
Spain	83.4
Israel	82.5
France	82.4
South Korea	82.4
Canada	81.9
Slovenia	81.3
United Kingdom	81.2
OECD Median Value	**81.2**
Costa Rica	79.6
United States	78.6
Poland	78.0
China	76.0
Mexico	75.4
Russia	71.8
India	68.4
South Africa	57.5

Source: OECD.

serious enough to seek urgent care in a hospital emergency room. The World Health Organization (WHO) reports that widening inequities across the world result in an estimated 100 million people being pushed into poverty every year when they are forced to pay out of pocket for health services.

The Constitution of the WHO envisions "the highest attainable standard of health as a fundamental right of every human being." Specifically, member-states must ensure access to timely, acceptable, and affordable healthcare of appropriate quality while providing for the underlying determinants of health, such as safe and potable water, sanitation, food, housing, health information and education, and gender equality. According to the WHO, the right to healthcare must be enjoyed without discrimination on the grounds of race, age, ethnicity, or any other status, and stakeholders (e.g., nongovernmental organizations) must be involved in all phases of programming—assessment, analysis, planning, implementation, monitoring, and evaluation. Unfortunately, many nations have a long way to go in achieving the WHO's vision of quality healthcare for all.

IMPACT ON URBAN HEALTH

People with limited access to quality healthcare face the highest risk of poor health outcomes, particularly people with low socioeconomic status, which is associated with increased risk of low birth weight, heart and lung disease, hypertension, arthritis, diabetes, autoimmune disorders, cancer, and illnesses linked to poor nutrition. Furthermore, studies have found that children in low-income families have worse health outcomes than children from high-income families. Urban health risks, already high in slum areas, may worsen as these areas expand. Roughly 40 percent of global urban growth is occurring in urban slum areas, and this trend is expected to continue as people move to cities from rural areas in search of jobs. Climate-change migration may force even more people into urban areas as drought ruins crops and sea level rise inundates coastal communities.

Even city residents with moderate and high incomes face greater risks of disease than people living in rural areas, particularly risks associated with the built environment. Air and water pollution, hazardous waste dump sites, automobile emissions, occupational exposures, and sound and light pollution are examples of environmental risks in the city that can lead to asthma, heart and lung disease, cancer, autoimmune diseases, mental stress, and other serious health problems. Additionally, infectious diseases can spread quickly in the urban environment, and food deserts (parts of cities void of grocery stores selling fresh fruits and vegetables and other wholesome foods) can lead to nutritional deficiencies. Climate change will exacerbate these risks by increasing urban smog levels and causing more frequent and longer-lasting heat waves.

Regardless of economic status, everyone in the city needs access to a high-quality healthcare system. This is especially important for children, who are at increased risk in urban areas for a variety of health conditions, including lead poisoning and asthma. Lead interferes with neurological development and is a particular problem in U.S. cities, such as Baltimore, Detroit, Cleveland, and parts of Philadelphia, which were once major manufacturing sites and where lead persists in the soil near the now-shuttered factories. Additionally, lead is sometimes found in domestic water supplies serviced by old lead pipes, and lead exposure can also occur when renovating old homes and other buildings with lead-based paint. In one 2016 study, 8.5 percent of Pennsylvania children were found to have elevated levels of lead in their blood. Urban children also suffer more than adults and their rural peers from asthma, a disease that causes repeated episodes of wheezing, breathlessness, chest tightness, and nighttime or early-morning coughing. Exposure to air pollution in urban areas can trigger asthma episodes or make episodes worse.

Access to quality healthcare in the city is critical for people with AIDS, which is caused by the human immunodeficiency virus (HIV). HIV is spread through certain body fluids and attacks the body's immune system, making it difficult for the body to fight infections and disease. AIDS is largely an urban disease, with most cases occurring in urban areas having populations of at least 500,000. (In the United States, urban areas in the Northeast have the highest number of AIDS cases per capita.) Globally, about 1 million people died from AIDS-related diseases in 2016, with the majority of new HIV infections occurring in sub-Saharan Africa. While prevention and treatment have improved, HIV remains a significant cause of death for certain populations. (Gay, bisexual, and other men who have sex with men are most at risk, but individuals can also be infected through heterosexual sex and by sharing needles.) In many countries, city health departments and clinics play a central role in treating AIDS and providing education and counseling.

Obtaining quality healthcare is also critical for fighting drug and alcohol abuse, especially the ongoing opioid epidemic. On average, 115 American die every day from a drug overdose involving opioids (including prescription opioids and illegal opioids like heroin and illicitly manufactured fentanyl), a death rate five times higher than in 1999, according to the Centers for Disease Control and Prevention. And globally, over 30 million people have drug-use disorders. In the United States, there are over 14,000 specialized drug treatment facilities, mostly in urban areas and often close to where drug abuse occurs. However, only a small percentage of people suffering from drug abuse and addiction problems seek help at these facilities or with other care providers. The reasons are complicated but have much to do with feelings of denial (refusal to recognize the substance abuse problem), shame (reluctance to admit to family members and others that they have a problem), and fear (concern about having the courage and determination to stick with a rigorous and difficult treatment-and-recovery program). In cities throughout the world, illicit drugs are associated with organized crime and gang violence.

About 88,000 Americans die annually from alcohol-related causes, representing the third-leading preventable cause of death in the United States. Additionally, alcohol-impaired driving results in around 10,000 deaths every year. Globally, alcohol consumption causes over 3 million deaths annually, almost 6 percent of all global deaths, and it contributes to over 200 types of diseases and injuries. Of course, the effects of alcoholism are not limited to the person who drinks. A 2018 study published in the *Journal of the American Medical Association* reported that many more American children than previously thought may be suffering from cognitive, behavioral, and physical developmental problems because of neurological damage occurring when their mother consumed alcohol while pregnant. Family members also suffer when a loved one loses a job, becomes habitually unreasonable or belligerent, and requires high medical expenses due to an alcohol problem. Alcoholism is similar to drug abuse, in that clinics and counseling services are commonly available in urban areas and many urban treatment facilities offer an array of related services not always available in rural areas, including detoxification centers and mental health services. The challenge is often not the availability of services but, as with drug abuse, getting alcoholics to use these services.

WHAT CITIES ARE DOING ABOUT HEALTHCARE ACCESS AND QUALITY

Although many healthcare programs and policies are managed at the federal and state levels of government, cities play a pivotal role in delivering healthcare services and increasing access to high-quality care. Additionally, cities often sponsor educational programming and financial assistance for underserved groups to encourage healthy lifestyles. Cities promote good health in other ways too, such as by investing in low-polluting public transportation systems, senior ride services to help older adults get to medical appointments, air and water pollution control regulations, green building initiatives, and climate-change-mitigation activities.

City health departments are usually at the forefront of urban healthcare services. While services differ from city to city, depending on local needs and funding, the following goals are common to many city health departments in the United States and other countries:

- Enforcing federal and state health regulations
- Monitoring and investigating health issues in the community
- Providing information about healthy choices
- Engaging the community in identifying and solving health challenges
- Assisting underserved groups in accessing health services
- Evaluating and improving health programs and interventions
- Collecting health and demographic data from the community

To achieve these goals, many cities have neighborhood clinics and treatment centers for a variety of health issues and needs, including family planning and pregnancy counseling, maternal and infant healthcare, immunizations, asthma treatment, cancer screening, lead poisoning prevention, drug and alcohol abuse treatment, tobacco cessation, teen pregnancy prevention, senior care, dental treatment, healthy food access, and education and treatment for AIDS and other sexually transmitted diseases. City hospitals and emergency rooms also provide treatment for more serious or urgent health problems. Some services may be low-cost or free to people with limited incomes. Additionally, a top priority of many cities is to reduce the infant mortality rate. Although infant mortality is falling, over 4 million deaths still occur worldwide during the first year of life, with the highest death rates occurring in Africa. Surprisingly, given the comparatively large amount of money spent on healthcare nationwide, the United States has a higher infant mortality rate (5.9 per 1,000 live births) than the OECD average (3.9 per 1,000 live births).

Many cities coordinate with existing social networks to improve healthcare and encourage those in need to seek treatment. One example is the National Urban Health Mission in India, which recruits volunteers and community workers to provide reproductive and women's health services in city slums, and a similar program in India trains volunteers to provide emotional support for patients receiving palliative care. Another example of leveraging social networks can be found in the Harlem neighborhood of New York City, where a group called City Health Works sends health "coaches" into the homes of low-income people with chronic illnesses, such as diabetes, hypertension, and asthma. The coaches build relationships with patients and help them access available resources. These and other community-based health programs have demonstrated improved health outcomes for patients while creating greater social cohesion within the community.

RECOMMENDATIONS FOR CITY DWELLERS

Prevention is key to maintaining health. For people concerned about healthcare access and affordability in their communities, remaining healthy should be their top priority. Some tips for remaining healthy while living in the city include the following:

- Take time to prepare healthy meals, and eat out less often, especially at fast food establishments.
- Get plenty of exercise, but stay indoors when the air pollution is bad. (In the United States, follow the AirNow Air Quality Index forecast.)
- Avoid unhealthy habits, such as smoking and drug and alcohol abuse.
- During flu season, avoid large crowds, wash hands frequently, and get a flu shot.
- Stay socially active and find relaxing ways to avoid stress (e.g., stay away from noisy areas and bright lights and avoid driving when the roads are congested).
- Remain alert for any unhealthy exposures or risks of injury at home and work.
- Take all common-sense precautions to avoid crime and violence in the city.
- Build a strong social support network among family members and friends.
- Get regular checkups at the doctor's office.

Having adequate health insurance coverage, including Medicare or Medicaid for older adults and others who qualify, can also help people stay healthy by increasing their access to the healthcare system. Unfortunately, many urban residents who are not provided health insurance by their employers cannot afford to purchase it on the open market, or they only can afford high-deductible policies where a large percentage of annual medical costs are paid out of pocket. Currently, about 9 percent of the U.S. population lacks any type of health insurance at all, and many of these people live in low-income urban areas. People finding themselves uninsured or underinsured (where insurance does not cover all of the medical costs) can find help at a community health center, and under a U.S. federal program, all people are entitled to care even if they cannot pay. A variety of other health services, including mental health support and drug and alcohol treatment, are available through city health departments and other agencies.

Healthcare access and quality are not problems of science or technology, but of public policy and allocation of resources. By speaking out in favor of better healthcare, voting for candidates who understand the healthcare challenges facing many urban dwellers, and even running for elected office as a pro-healthcare candidate, people living in the city can help improve healthcare access and the quality of life for everyone in their neighborhoods.

CITY SPOTLIGHT: DELHI—REFORMING THE DELIVERY OF URBAN HEALTH SERVICES

Access to quality healthcare in Delhi is challenging for the city's poor residents, especially the multitude of slum dwellers and migrants from even-poorer parts of the country. But a network of people's health clinics is proving that decent healthcare need not be limited to those who are well off.

India is a land of contrasts in many ways, including the quality and availability of healthcare. The country is home to some of the leading hospitals in the world, renowned medical teaching institutions, and outstanding medical professionals. At the same time, many people, especially the poor, receive low-quality medical services, if they can access the medical system at all. To address these healthcare disparities, a new network of people's clinics has sprung up in Delhi, India's capital city.

Delhi, a vast metropolis having a population of around 26 million, comprises 11 districts, one of which is New Delhi, where the national capital is located. (Delhi is the world's third-largest metropolitan area.) Like the rest of India, healthcare in Delhi suffers from low government funding and a high prevalence of communicable diseases, such as tuberculosis and measles. Also, there is a growing threat from noncommunicable diseases, including diabetes, hypertension, and cancer. Because public hospitals and other public health facilities are often overcrowded with long waits for service, and because the quality of healthcare provided is sometimes questionable, most people prefer private medical care if they can afford it. But for the multitude of poor people, including the 10 percent of Delhi's population living in slums, going to a public health facility is their only option.

To address these inequities, the mohalla community health clinic concept has recently taken root. (The clinics are referred to as "mohallas," or more simply, "the people's clinics.") The mohalla concept grew out of the successful mobile medical unit program, where mobile vans provide basic healthcare services to underserved neighborhoods, often in slum areas. When contemplating expansion of this program, Delhi government officials struggled with several obstacles to providing better service, such as the complexity of purchasing and maintaining a large number of new vehicles, the difficulty of recruiting qualified drivers and medical staff, and the challenge of keeping mobile units stocked with medicines and other supplies. And driving the units over the rough and sometimes hazardous roads in some parts of town was another concern. In search of a better solution, mohallas were born.

The main idea behind the mohalla clinics is to provide free healthcare to people of limited means by placing up to 1,000 health clinics in neighborhoods where basic healthcare and diagnostic services are most needed, and by locating the clinics within walking distance for people needing care. By locating free clinics in neighborhoods, it was reasoned that people would come who otherwise may not seek medical attention until their condition becomes serious enough to require hospitalization. The clinics were designed to provide basic outpatient services, including first aid, maternal and child healthcare, immunization, family planning, counseling, and if needed, referral to specialists. Between 80 and 90 percent of the health concerns of people in these areas are related to minor ailments like fevers, headaches, infections, and skin rashes that can be easily handled by the mohallas, thereby freeing staff time in hospitals and other health clinics to address more serious problems.

Currently, there are over 150 mohalla clinics, and more are in the works. The clinics have been very popular, seeing an average of 70–100 patients per day, and in 2016, the first year of operation for most of the existing clinics, there were over 1.5 million patient visits. One early success story concerns a serious outbreak of dengue and chikungunya diseases, when the mohalla clinics provided many initial examinations and laboratory tests, preventing thousands of patients from jamming into hospital waiting rooms. Overall, patients report being highly satisfied with the mohalla's quick check-in process, limited wait times, fast turnarounds on test analyses, and the absence of bills and paperwork. Nevertheless, the mohalla program has a long way to go to achieve the goal of 1,000 free clinics in Delhi, and ongoing delays associated with land allotment issues, finances, and government infighting still need to be resolved.

One exciting technological innovation in use at the mohallas is the Swasthya Slate, a small, portable diagnostic tool that connects to the Internet through a cell phone or tablet computer and can (1) perform up to 33 diagnostic tests within about 45 minutes; (2) create an electronic health file for the patient; and (3) send out appointment and vaccination reminders. The device can test for malaria, dengue, hepatitis, HIV, and typhoid, and it can check blood pressure, blood sugar, heart rate, blood hemoglobin, urine protein, and glucose. Best of all, it requires minimal training and costs very little to operate.

The Swasthya Slate was developed by Kanav Kahol, a biomedical engineer and researcher in the United States who became frustrated at the lack of interest within the U.S. medical establishment in reducing diagnostic costs. However, he found great interest in India, and the device is also gaining popularity in other developing nations. Despite its success in Delhi, some issues remain, such as slow or intermittent Internet service, periods when the electricity is out, problems sharing electronic patient records with hospitals and health clinics, and patients who insist on handwritten prescriptions. (The device manages all data electronically, including prescriptions.) A newer version of the Swasthya Slate, HealthCube, is now on the market.

While not a perfect solution to the unmet healthcare needs of Delhi, the mohalla clinics have been very well received, causing health professionals to rethink healthcare delivery across all of India. In particular, the clinics may serve as a workable model for strengthening primary healthcare and eliminating inequities for the country's poorest inhabitants, and the mohalla experiment in Delhi may eventually lead the way to universal healthcare for all. Evidence continues to build regarding the value of the mohalla program to the nation, including use data demonstrating that nearly half of the first-time users of the clinics were visiting a government healthcare facility for the first time in their lives.

Indoor Air Quality

When discussing air pollution, the first image that comes to mind for many people is a tall smokestack beside a dirty industrial manufacturing facility, or perhaps the exhaust from hundreds of automobiles on a busy freeway. But you may be surprised that air pollution inside a building—indoor air pollution—can be as big a threat to public health in a city as outside air pollution. When air pollution levels inside buildings are high enough to affect health, we say that the *quality* of the indoor air is threatened.

Indoor air pollution levels can be as much as 5 times higher than outside air pollution in some urban buildings, and cases have been documented where indoor levels were 100 times higher. Indoor air quality is a serious public health concern because most adults spend about 90 percent of their time indoors (e.g., working in an office building or factory, eating out at restaurants, shopping, relaxing at home, and sleeping). Children spend more time outside than adults, but even so, the majority of a typical child's time is spent indoors, usually at school and home.

How does inside air become polluted? There are a number of potential sources of indoor air pollution in a building, including:

- **Combustion appliances.** These are devices used for warmth, cooking, or decorative purposes that burn fuel, such as coal, oil, natural and liquefied petroleum gas, kerosene, and wood. Ranges, furnaces, space heaters, water heaters, and fireplaces are common examples of these devices. Old or improperly operated combustion appliances can sometimes release carbon monoxide (CO) and other pollutants into the surrounding air.

- **Tobacco products.** This includes (1) cigarette, cigar, and pipe smoke; (2) secondhand smoke, which is smoke that you may inhale that is emitted by others who are smoking in your vicinity; and (3) thirdhand smoke, which is smoke residue that collects on walls and other surfaces and later becomes airborne, often reacting with other indoor air pollutants to create a toxic mix of chemicals. There is growing concern about secondhand exposure to flavoring agents, formaldehyde, glycols, nicotine, nitrosamines, and other chemicals exhaled by e-cigarette smokers.

- **Building materials and furnishings.** Many building materials, such as wallboard, composite wood products (e.g., plywood, particleboard, and fiberboard), insulation, carpeting, upholstery, and paint and other surface coatings, contain volatile organic compounds and other chemicals that can contribute indoor air pollution. Renovation projects involving older homes and buildings sometimes disturb asbestos insulation and lead-containing paint, resulting in asbestos fibers and lead particles being released into the indoor air.

- **Household cleaners, personal care products, insecticides, and hobby supplies.** These products contain a wide variety of chemicals, such as disinfectants, pesticides, solvents, and glues, which can become airborne, particularly when dispensed using a spray can or bottle. A recent analysis of data from the European Community Respiratory Health Survey found that regular exposure to cleaning products may significantly affect lung function and accelerate the rate of lung function decline that occurs with age.

- **Biological substances.** Mold and mildew, viruses and bacteria, and pet dander are examples of biological substances that may become airborne inside a building. Additionally, the protein in rat and mice urine, a potent allergen, can become airborne after it dries. If not properly maintained, mechanical air handling systems can sometime present ideal conditions for the growth of mold and mildew, which may subsequently be distributed throughout the building when the systems are operated.

- **Outdoor air pollutants.** Outdoor air pollution, including ozone, fine particles, radon, and agricultural chemicals, can enter a building through open doors and windows, ventilation systems, and cracks in walls and foundations. Pollens and other allergy-causing contaminants can also enter a building from the outside.

Some specific examples of pollutants that can adversely affect indoor air quality are listed in Table 12.

The modern, energy-efficient buildings found in many urban areas can sometimes make indoor air pollution worse because they are tightly sealed to prevent heat from leaking to the outside air in the winter and warm air from entering the building in the summer. If these buildings lack good

Table 12   Examples of Indoor Air Pollutants

Pollutant	Typical Source
Acetic acid	X-ray equipment, caulking compounds
Formaldehyde	Insulation, plywood, particle board, paneling, carpeting, fabric adhesives, tobacco smoke
Inorganic gases—ammonia, hydrogen sulfide, sulfur dioxide, and others	Window cleaners, acid drain cleaners, tobacco smoke, blueprint equipment, gas furnaces and appliances, engine exhaust
Microbials—viruses, fungi, mold, bacteria, pollen, dander, and mites	Air-handling systems, cooling towers, humidifiers, water-damaged materials, plants, food and food products
Nitrogen oxide	Gas furnaces and appliances, welding operations, engine exhaust, tobacco smoke
Ozone	Copy machines, electrostatic air cleaners, outside air
Radon	Decay of radioactive elements found in some soil and rock and in some building materials, including brick, gypsum, and concrete
Secondhand tobacco smoke	People who smoke tobacco products indoors, such as cigarettes, cigars, and pipes
Volatile organic compounds—trichloroethylene, benzene, toluene, methyl ethyl ketone, alcohols, acrolein, and others	Paint, cleaning products and disinfectants, mothballs, glues, photocopiers, caulking materials, pesticides, cosmetics and other personal products

Source: EPA.

ventilation, indoor air pollutants can increase to levels much higher than in the outside air, and if humidity also builds up, some indoor pollutants can become even more hazardous. Many newer buildings address this problem by incorporating devices such as energy recovery ventilators, which are designed to conserve energy while still allowing a reasonable amount of ventilation. Also, the latest high-efficiency furnaces are typically designed to draw in ventilation air from the outside. (See the "Green Buildings and Sustainable Development" entry for more information on air quality inside energy-efficient "green" buildings.)

About half the world's population lives in rural towns and villages, where they often cook indoors with simple stoves or open hearths (e.g., fireplaces) fueled by wood, coal, dung, or agricultural residue. Because of poor ventilation in their homes, which sometimes comprise just a single room or two with a dirt floor, smoke can build up to high levels, resulting in serious health concerns. In some homes, concentrations of fine particulates, CO, and other air pollutants can exceed safe levels by up to 100 times.

This is not just a rural problem, though; some of the world's largest cities are in developing nations, and up to 25 percent of households there still rely on indoor cookstoves to prepare their meals. The World Health Organization (WHO) estimates that every year, about 3.8 million people worldwide die prematurely from exposure to household air pollutants, mainly from indoor cooking. The risks are greatest among poor women and children, who often spend more time at home, where they inhale copious amounts of smoke and soot. Air pollution—both indoor and outdoor—represents the world's greatest environment health risk.

IMPACT ON URBAN HEALTH

Good indoor air quality is important because irritants in the air can diminish our productivity at work and performance at school. More important, some indoor air pollutants can affect our health, sometimes causing serious illness. Symptoms associated with poor indoor air quality can include:

- allergic reactions
- irritation of the eye, nose, throat, and skin
- coughing and sneezing
- dizziness
- headache and fatigue

- nausea
- shortness of breath
- sinus congestion

Additionally, exposure to indoor air pollution can cause serious illnesses, like Legionnaires' disease and lung cancer.

Unfortunately, indoor air quality problems can be subtle and often difficult to diagnose, due in part to the presence of other factors that may aggravate or cause similar symptoms. For example, having a cold or the flu can cause symptoms that mimic some indoor air pollution symptoms, inadequate lighting or air conditioning at work or school can cause headaches and fatigue, and stress from a heavy workload or personal situation at home can make us more susceptible to disease. Furthermore, some individuals are more sensitive to indoor air pollution due to preexisting conditions such as asthma or allergies, respiratory disease, or a weakened immune system caused by illness or medical treatment. Building occupants with heart disease may be more susceptible to CO pollution, and those who wear contact lenses may be more sensitive to indoor air contaminants that irritate the eyes. Children are more susceptible to indoor air pollutants because their bodies are still developing, and they breathe more air in proportion to their body weight than adults.

Some health effects associated with poor indoor air quality appears quickly and can be effectively treated by eliminating exposure to the pollution source. For example, offensive cleaning products or building materials can be replaced and mold or mildew in an air-handling system can be removed. However, other health problems that are more serious, like heart and respiratory disease and cancer, may not appear until years after exposure or only after repeated exposures over a long period. Thus, even if no symptoms have occurred in your home, school, or workplace, it is a good idea to prevent indoor air pollution anyway, to avoid future health issues.

Researchers have found that children, older adults, minorities, low-income people, and tribes and indigenous people are sometimes disproportionately affected by indoor pollutants, such as asthma triggers, secondhand smoke, mold, and radon. This means that these people are exposed to higher levels of indoor pollution compared with other segments of the population, often due to socioeconomic conditions that result in reduced access to homes, schools, and workplaces that have healthy indoor air. The term "environmental justice" refers to efforts to eliminate disparities in exposure to environmental pollution, including indoor air quality.

Exposure disparities in urban populations are usually best addressed on a local scale by cities and communities, although some nonprofit organizations and government agencies provide consultation and guidance.

One of the most common indoor air quality complaints concerns sick building syndrome (SBS), a term used to describe the headache, nausea, fatigue, and other ill health symptoms that building occupants sometimes experience while inside the building. SBS is most common in office buildings, but it can also occur in apartments, schools, and other buildings with multiple occupants. The presence of SBS in a particular building is often difficult to confirm, but if the symptoms subside or completely disappear after occupants leave the building, the cause of the discomfort is assumed to be something inside. The symptoms may be limited to a specific room or area of the building, or they may be reported throughout the building, and they may or may not occur seasonally. To be considered SBS, health professionals typically look for symptoms among a group of occupants rather than one or two isolated cases.

Inadequate building ventilation is thought to contribute to many cases of SBS because without enough ventilation, air pollutants can increase to levels that adversely affect health. The air pollutants causing SBS may originate inside the building, such as from carpeting, wall paint, particle board, pesticides, office machines, air fresheners, dust mites, and even marking pens. Alternatively, indoor air pollution may be caused by outside air contaminants, including pollen, that have permeated the building. SBS can also be caused by mold and other microbial pathogens, particularly when they grow and accumulate in air-handling equipment and in water-damaged wallboard, ceiling tile, carpeting, and insulation. Odors, stagnant air, thermal gradients, high humidity, poor lighting, office noise, and inadequate sanitary and cleaning practices may also contribute to SBS symptoms.

Legionnaires' disease is another air quality health condition associated with buildings, although it differs from SBS in that it can be attributed to a specific pathogen in the building. This disease is a type of pneumonia (i.e., lung infection) caused by the *Legionella* bacteria, which can grow and spread in showers, faucets, and mechanical devices, such as plumbing systems, water tanks and heaters, and commercial air conditioning units. (Home and automobile air conditioners are not at risk for *Legionella* propagation because they do not use water.) Hot tubs that are not properly drained after each use can also harbor *Legionella*. When operating a shower, faucet, or mechanical device containing water, small droplets of water can become airborne. If these droplets are contaminated with the *Legionella* bacteria, and if you inhale the droplets, you are at risk of becoming sick with Legionnaires' disease. Inhalation exposure can also occur by the aspiration of water into the trachea and lungs as we drink *Legionella*-contaminated water from a glass or water fountain. A related condition caused by the *Legionella* bacteria, Pontiac fever, is a milder infection that does not involve pneumonia.

In addition to SBS and Legionnaires' disease, building managers need to take precautions to prevent occupants from being exposed to other pathogenic agents, such as *Norovirus*, which is a highly contagious virus causing acute gastroenteritis. Cases of people contracting this virus are more common in enclosed areas, such as day-care centers, nursing homes, schools, and college dormitories, and outbreaks typically occur during the winter months, perhaps because building ventilation is reduced to conserve heat. *Norovirus* is also implicated in many food-related illnesses, and it is particularly notorious for causing outbreaks on cruise ships.

Another indoor air pollution concern for city buildings is CO poisoning. CO gases are emitted when fuels are combusted in appliances, such as ranges, furnaces, space heaters, water heaters, and fireplaces. If the appliance is used in an enclosed area with poor ventilation, the CO gases can build up to dangerous levels. On average, over 400 Americans die each year from unintentional CO poisoning not related to fires, more than 20,000 are rushed to emergency rooms, and over 4,000 are hospitalized. The WHO reports that CO exposure remains one of the leading causes of unintentional and suicidal poisonings, causing a large number of deaths every year.

Radon is a well-known problem in many urban areas, causing over 20,000 lung cancer deaths in the United States annually, according to the U.S. Environmental Protection Agency (EPA), and the WHO believes that radon exposure is responsible for tens of thousands of lung cancer deaths occurring globally every year. It represents the second-leading cause of lung cancer in the United States, second only to tobacco smoking. Radon is a radioactive gas that forms naturally from the decay of radioactive elements found in some soil, rock, brick, gypsum, concrete, and other building materials. When city buildings incorporate these radon-emitting materials, or when buildings are built on top of soil containing radioactive elements, radon gas can enter the structure and concentrate in living and working spaces, potentially building up to levels high enough to increase the risk of lung cancer. While radon can accumulate in all types of buildings, the greatest exposure often occurs at home because we spend the majority of our time there.

The hazards of smoking are well established, but many people are not aware that being exposed to secondhand or thirdhand smoke inside a building can also be hazardous to your health, particularly if you occupy a poorly ventilated space with a smoker. Of the over 7 million deaths occurring globally each year that are attributed to tobacco use, about 900,000 are among nonsmokers exposed to secondhand smoke. Researchers have identified more than 7,000 chemicals in tobacco smoke, at least 250 of which are harmful to human health, and over 50 are known carcinogens. Because of these concerns, as well as general complaints from nonsmokers about having to smell tobacco smoke while at work or in public spaces, many building owners and municipalities prohibit smoking inside buildings or limit smoking to well-ventilated designated areas. The WHO states unequivocally that there is no safe level of exposure to secondhand tobacco smoke, and the EPA has concluded that "exposure to secondhand smoke can cause lung cancer in adults who do not smoke."

WHAT CITIES ARE DOING ABOUT INDOOR AIR QUALITY

Few cities have offices or experts dedicated to indoor air quality, but many cities do address indoor air quality through zoning laws, construction permits, and local ordinances. For example, landlords may be required to keep buildings clean, sanitary, and pest-free, and building contractors may need to meet the latest "best practices" for heating, air conditioning, ventilation, building materials, and alarms (e.g., smoke and CO detectors). Many cities prohibit smoking in public spaces and specify procedures for renovating or demolishing old buildings containing lead paint or asbestos insulation. In larger cities, local health departments and environmental agencies may provide advice and recommendations on improving indoor air quality, perform inspections, and issue citations when violations of city codes occur.

When confronting an indoor air quality problem, city health and environmental officials ordinarily first try to identify the source of the problem while assessing whether poor ventilation is a contributing factor. An approach that is sometimes recommended is to install an air cleaner (also called an "air purifier"), which can range in size from a tabletop model to an expensive whole-house or entire-building system. Some air cleaners are

effective in removing particles from the air, but most air cleaners are ineffective in removing gaseous pollutants. The most effective air cleaners have
high-efficiency filters and can handle a large volume of air. On the other
hand, less expensive tabletop models often have limited effectiveness, except
in confined areas. Also, air cleaners, regardless of size and efficiency, may
not satisfactorily protect people with high sensitivities to particular sources
or allergens.

Lately, there has been some interest in using indoor plants as air cleaners, and some modern urban buildings incorporate houseplants and other
greenery for this purpose. Having indoor plants helps create a pleasant work
environment, but the EPA reports that there is currently no evidence that a
reasonable number of houseplants can remove significant quantities of
pollutants in homes and offices. Also, the EPA does not recommend using
air cleaners marketed to reduce radon exposure, concluding that "the
effectiveness of these devices is uncertain because they only partially
remove the radon decay products and do not diminish the amount of radon
entering the home." Some manufacturers market indoor air cleaners that
generate ozone, which they claim can be highly effective in reducing a
variety of indoor air pollutants. However, the EPA has found that the ozone
concentrations produced by some ozone-based air cleaners can exceed
health standards, and that at concentrations that do not exceed health standards, these devices are generally ineffective in reducing indoor air
pollution.

RECOMMENDATIONS FOR CITY DWELLERS

Here are some common-sense steps that everyone should take to reduce
the risk of illness from indoor air pollution:

- Ensure that your home or business has adequate ventilation, particularly during the winter months when windows are shut while fuel-
  burning appliances like space heaters and woodstoves are in use.

- Use only household cleaners and personal care products that are manufactured from nontoxic substances. Restrict hobby activities using
  glues, chemicals, and paints to well-ventilated areas. Avoid using pesticides by regularly sweeping and vacuuming food particles that can
  attract pests. When necessary, use only nonchemical methods of pest
  control.

- Test your home or business for radon, and if found at significant levels, take appropriate remedial action to reduce your exposure. (Inexpensive, do-it-yourself test kits are available.)

- Remove any standing water (e.g., in humidifier reservoirs and drain pans), and replace water-damaged materials, including wallboard, ceiling tile, carpeting, and insulation.

- If building a home, select materials and furnishings that are made of environmentally friendly materials that do not emit toxic gases into the surrounding air. If renovating an old home, check with experts to be sure that there is no lead paint or asbestos present. If these materials are found, consult with a trained and qualified contractor to determine whether these materials should be removed or sealed in place.

- CO monitors should be installed outside each sleeping area and in areas where CO could leak from a combustion appliance. If you have a furnace, water heater, gas range, or any other appliances that use gas, oil, or coal, have it inspected annually, and refrain from using appliances inside your home, basement, or garage that emit CO gases. It is always a mistake to run the engine of your car or truck inside a garage, even if the garage door is open.

- Stay away from people who smoke, and never allow smoking inside your home. (Among the world's 1.1 billion smokers, up to half will die from lung cancer and other illnesses directly caused by smoking, according to the WHO, and many more will die from exposure to secondhand and thirdhand smoke.)

Poor ventilation is believed to be associated with SBS about half the time. Ventilation can be improved by adjusting or replacing mechanical systems and regularly performing preventive maintenance (e.g., cleaning ducts and dampers and changing air filters). When ventilation systems are in use, air quality can be improved by adding air treatment (e.g., carbon filters), locating outside air intakes away from potential air pollution sources (e.g., garages and roadways), and ensuring temperature and humidity standards are consistently maintained. (Humidity should generally be below 60 percent to discourage microbial growth.)

While indoor diseases like SBS are mainly air quality issues, research suggests that synergistic effects involving stress may result in symptoms that otherwise may not be present. A number of conditions can lead to occupational stress, including tight deadlines, a noisy work environment, poor work area lighting and temperature control, eye strain, ergonomic problems from computer work, work/life balance issues, and communication problems with coworkers or supervisors. Stress can also result from personal problems at home. Thus, in certain circumstances, stress management might be considered along with other measures to address symptoms.

It is estimated that about 1 of every 10 people with Legionnaires' disease will die due to complications from pneumonia. Thus, individuals developing symptoms of pneumonia should seek medical attention immediately. To help diagnose the problem, the doctor may ask if the individual might have been exposed to the *Legionella* bacteria or used a hot tub, spent nights away from home, or stayed in a hospital during the past two weeks.

People in developing countries, particularly in Southeast Asia, the Western Pacific, and Africa, need to be cautious about the use of indoor cookstoves and fires. The WHO, Global Alliance for Clean Cookstoves, and other international organizations are addressing this global health issue by developing cleaner cookstoves and teaching local people about techniques to reduce their exposure to hazardous air contaminants, such as burning cleaner fuels and improving ventilation. Electrification programs in remote villages, sometimes using solar power, have also helped reduced dependence on dirty fuels. Behavioral changes have been beneficial too, such as teaching people to dry wood before using it so that the wood burns cleaner, producing less indoor pollution.

Infectious Diseases

Infectious diseases are caused by pathogenic microorganisms, including certain types of bacteria, viruses, fungi, and parasites. (Sometimes we call these microorganisms "germs.") Urban areas are conducive to the spread of infectious diseases due to high population density and likelihood of exposure to others who may be infected (e.g., when riding a bus or shopping in a busy market). Good sanitation can also be a problem in urban areas, where trash in vacant lots and alleys may harbor rats and other vermin. Additionally, the puddling of rainwater in yards and on streets can provide an ideal breeding environment for disease-carrying mosquitoes. Infectious diseases are particularly rampant in some of the larger cities of developing nations, where the residents of shantytown and slum areas suffer from poor sanitation and limited access to healthcare, and where illicit drug use may be prevalent. More people die worldwide from infectious diseases than from any other single cause.

Two infectious diseases that we are all too familiar with are the common cold and the flu, and many of us have also experienced strep throat, stomach flu (gastroenteritis), and infections of the middle ear or urinary tract. The National Notifiable Diseases Surveillance System tracks a number of other infectious diseases present in the United States, including campylobacteriosis, chlamydia trachomatis infection, coccidioidomycosis (valley fever), cryptosporidiosis, giardiasis, gonorrhea, human immunodeficiency virus (HIV), invasive pneumococcal disease, Lyme disease, mumps, pertussis (whooping cough), salmonellosis, shigellosis, syphilis, tuberculosis, varicella (chickenpox), and Zika. These and other infectious diseases found throughout the world can cause a range of symptoms, from mild discomfort and fever to serious complications and even death. Table 13 summarizes the types of pathogenic microorganisms that cause infectious diseases.

There are four mechanisms by which infections can spread: (1) person-to-person, such as being exposed to germs from someone who is coughing or sneezing, or through kissing or sexual contact; (2) mother-to-unborn-child, such as germs that pass through the placenta or germs in the vagina that are transmitted to the baby during birth; (3) animal-to-person, including being bitten or scratched by an infected animal or by handling animal waste; and (4) indirect contact, such as exposure to germs that linger on countertops and doorknobs or that are present in contaminated food and water.

An infectious disease that can spread from person to person or by way of a vector, such as a mosquito or tick, is called a "communicable disease." All communicable diseases are infectious, but not all infectious diseases are communicable. For example, noncommunicable infections can be caused by toxins found naturally in the environment, such as the *Clostridium tetani* bacteria found in soil, dust, and manure that causes tetanus (sometimes called "lockjaw").

Zoonotic diseases are infectious diseases of animals that can be transmitted to humans, and surprisingly, up to 60 percent of all infectious diseases in humans are zoonotic in origin. Several examples are Lyme disease and Rocky Mountain spotted fever (transmitted by ticks), malaria and West Nile virus (transmitted by mosquitoes), and *Escherichia coli* and *Salmonella* infections (from handling infected animals or eating contaminated animal food products). Also, it is well known that we can contract rabies from cats, dogs, bats, and other animals found in urban areas. Anthrax, another type of zoonotic disease, can be contracted by touching infected animals and contaminated animal products, although anthrax outbreaks affecting humans are rare. Urban expansion, along with climate change, is expected to result in an increase in zoonotic diseases as animal habitats change and wildlife come into more frequent contact with humans.

A seminal event in the history of infectious diseases in urban areas was the discovery by John Snow (1813–1858) that cholera was a contagious disease spread by contaminated drinking water. (We now know that it can also spread by contaminated food.) By studying cholera deaths in London households supplied by two different water companies—one company supplying clean water and the other contaminated water—Snow proved that consumption of the contaminated water resulted in a higher risk of

Table 13   Pathogenic Microorganisms Causing Infectious Diseases

Microorganism	Description
Bacteria	Complex, single-celled organisms that can reproduce on their own and are responsible for a number of common illnesses, such as strep throat, urinary tract infection, and tuberculosis. Bacteria have been around for over 3 billion years, and they are capable of surviving in extreme environments, including intense heat and cold. Not all bacteria are harmful, and some can even be useful. For example, *Lactobacillus acidophilus* is a harmless bacteria that resides in your intestines, helping to digest food, destroy harmful organisms, and provide nutrients.
Viruses	Submicroscopic infective agents that differ from bacteria in that they can only grow and reproduce in living cells. Viruses can cause a variety of illnesses, ranging from influenza and the common cold to AIDS, a potentially life-threatening illness caused by HIV. Antibiotics that have proved to be effective on bacteria have no effect on viruses.
Fungi	A group of eukaryotic organisms that reproduce by means of spores. Fungi are present in soil, air, and water, and although most species are of little concern, several types of fungi can cause diseases, including coccidioidomycosis, ringworm, and athlete's foot. Thrush, an infection of the mouth and throat mainly affecting infants and children, is caused by a yeast called *Candida albicans*. A number of harmless fungi are common in our diets (e.g., mushrooms and the blue/green veins in some cheeses).
Parasites	Types of organisms (e.g., protozoa, helminths, and ectoparasites) that take nourishment from a host they live on or within. Parasite infections can result in serious illnesses, such as malaria, which is caused by a parasite transmitted by mosquitos. The CDC has targeted five neglected parasitic infections as priorities for public action: Chagas disease, cysticercosis, toxocariasis, toxoplasmosis, and trichomoniasis.

cholera. Later, in the twentieth century, infectious diseases declined pre-cipitously in many parts of the world due to improved sanitation and hygiene, the discovery of antibiotics, and universal vaccination programs for children. This decline was aided by the creation of many local and regional health departments and environmental agencies that implemented vaccina-tion programs, as well as a number of crucial disease prevention initiatives aimed at improving water quality, sewage disposal, pest control, food handling, and other sanitation and hygiene practices.

IMPACT ON URBAN HEALTH

Infectious diseases can spread quickly in an urban environment, caus-ing a number of health concerns that vary depending on the infecting organ-ism and the type of disease. Symptoms often include fever, fatigue, diarrhea, coughing, and muscle aches, and while some infections will clear up with rest at home, others may require hospitalization for life-threatening conditions. City residents may be more susceptible to contracting infectious diseases if their immune systems are under stress due to illness or to medi-cations that suppress the immune system. Children and older adults are often at greater risk of infection, as are people whose bodies may be weak-ened from physical or emotional stress or urban pollution. Complications from infectious diseases are unusual, but they do occur. For example, pneu-monia, AIDS, and meningitis infections can become life-threatening, and some infections have been associated with increased risk of cancer. Other infections become silent for decades, only to reappear in the future, as in the case of childhood chicken pox causing shingles later in life.

A growing concern for the treatment of bacteria-related infections is anti-biotic resistance, which has resulted in illnesses once treatable with antibi-otics now becoming more of a threat to public health. In particular, some illnesses, such as gonorrhea, pneumonia, and tuberculosis, are becoming more complex, longer-lasting, and difficult to treat, requiring stronger and more expensive drugs. According to the World Health Organization (WHO), antibiotic resistance is one of the world's greatest threats to global health, and the U.S. Centers for Disease Control and Prevention (CDC) reports that over 2 million Americans become infected with antibiotic-resistant bacte-ria every year, many dying from their infections. Several reasons for the increase in antibiotic-resistant bacteria are the overuse and misuse of these drugs, improper prescribing, widespread presence of antibiotics in foods derived from animals, and a reduced number of new antibiotics coming on the market.

The most frequently seen infection is the common cold, which is a viral infection of the nose and throat. Anyone can get a cold, but if you live in a city, chances are you are more likely to be exposed to the germs. Although many types of viruses can cause a cold, it is almost always harmless, other than the discomfort we feel while the infection runs its course. It is not unusual for both children and adults to have one or several colds annually, usually during the colder months of the year. If you spend significant time around people at work or school, you are more likely to be exposed to the viruses that cause a cold, and smoking also can increase your risk of catching a cold by damaging lung cells and weakening the immune system. When complications occur, they typically involve ear infections, strep throat, or pneumonia, and a cold also can trigger asthma attacks.

Another common viral infection, especially in urban environments where germs can spread easily, is influenza (i.e., the flu). Influenza is associated with various symptoms, including fever, aching muscles, chills and sweats, headache, cough, fatigue, nasal congestion, and sore throat, and although it usually resolves on its own, serious cases can cause death. The CDC reports that influenza typically causes between 9 and 36 million illnesses and between 12,000 and 56,000 deaths annually in the United States. While anyone can develop complications from influenza, at the greatest risk are children and older adults, residents of nursing homes and long-term-care facilities, pregnant women and women up to two weeks postpartum, people with weakened immune systems and chronic illnesses, and people who are very obese. The most serious complication, pneumonia, can be deadly. Others include bronchitis, asthma flare-ups, heart problems, and ear infections. Annual vaccinations can prevent the flu or cause it to be less severe.

One virus that has gained considerable attention recently is *Norovirus*, which causes an estimated 20 million acute gastroenteritis cases in the United States every year. (Only the common cold, and in some years the flu, are more prevalent.) This highly contagious virus causes acute gastroenteritis, which is inflammation of the stomach or intestines or both, leading to diarrhea, vomiting, dehydration, nausea, stomach pain, and sometimes fever, headache, and body aches. In the United States, about half of all food-related illnesses are caused by the *Norovirus*. Enclosed areas, such as daycare centers, nursing homes, schools, and college dormitories, are particularly conducive to the spread of the *Norovirus*, and most outbreaks occur during the winter months. *Norovirus* is particularly notorious for out-breaks on cruise ships, where it is responsible for over 90 percent of diar-rheal disease cases. Currently, there are no medicines that are effective in treating *Norovirus* infections, and because there are many different types of *Norovirus*, being infected in the past and building up a resistance may not be protective against future infections from different strains of the virus.

A common source of infection in urban areas is contaminated food, including beverages. Globally, over 400,000 people die annually from dis-eases associated with contaminated food, and in the United States, one in six Americans become ill from eating foods contaminated with bacteria, viruses, or parasites. Some of these foodborne diseases are caused by the pathogen itself, while others are caused by the human body's reaction to the organism or the pathogenic toxin that it creates. Examples of foodborne diseases are botulism, hepatitis A, *Norovirus* infection, salmonellosis, and shigellosis.

Hospitals, clinics, nursing homes, and rehabilitation centers are often plagued by healthcare-associated infections (HAIs), which are infections that patients acquire while being treated for another condition. Healthcare staff can acquire HAIs as well as patients. Most HAIs are caused by micro-organisms that are common in the general population, where they typi-cally cause mild symptoms or no symptoms at all. But in a healthcare setting, where the patient is undergoing treatment and the immune system may be compromised, exposure to these common microorganisms can be much more serious, sometimes resulting in complications, a prolonged hos-pital stay, and even death. The most common HAIs are urinary tract, sur-gical site, and bloodstream infections and pneumonia, and infection rates tend to be higher among patients who are older, have underlying diseases, or are undergoing diagnostic and therapeutic interventions. The WHO esti-mates that every year, hundreds of millions of patients around the world are affected by HAIs, especially in low- and middle-income countries. In the United States, about 1 in every 25 hospital patients acquires an HAI, costing the U.S. healthcare system billions of dollars each year.

Over 800 million people live in urban slums, representing about one-third of the world's urban population. The overcrowded and unsanitary con-ditions in these areas facilitate the spread of many infectious diseases, including cholera, dengue fever, hepatitis, malaria, pneumonia, and tuber-culosis. The residents of urban slums also often suffer from diarrhea and are at high risk from heat waves, cold weather, and severe storms. Infec-tious diseases, combined with poor sanitation, polluted drinking water and air, inadequate diet, exposure to the weather, long hours of physical exertion at menial jobs, and limited healthcare options, result in widespread suffering in slum areas, particularly for children and older adults, who are often the most vulnerable to infectious diseases.

WHAT CITIES ARE DOING ABOUT INFECTIOUS DISEASES

City health departments are playing a leading role in controlling infectious diseases. For example, most health departments in large cities provide communicable and infectious disease surveillance programs, child and adult immunization services, screening and treatment for infectious diseases like tuberculosis and HIV/AIDS, food service establishment inspections, food safety education, and school and day-care-center inspections, and many health departments in smaller cities also offer some of these services. In addition, some health departments provide laboratory services or coordinate laboratory analyses with state laboratories. Health departments consider tracking and responding to outbreaks of infectious diseases like influenza among their highest priorities.

Larger health departments may have epidemiologists, toxicologists, and physicians on staff who can conduct detailed studies into the incidence, distribution, health effects, and control of infectious diseases. Additionally, some health departments may have professionals who are specifically trained to prevent or control the spread infectious diseases. Their activities may include (1) organizing clinics to provide childhood or influenza vaccinations or deliver educational programs and materials on sexually transmitted diseases; (2) assessing trends to determine priorities for future interventions; (3) working with community groups to offer health promotion and disease prevention activities; and (4) providing education and healthcare management for people at higher risk for certain infections.

Although infectious diseases can spread quickly through urban areas, cities are often well prepared to fight infectious diseases because of their infectious disease surveillance, control, and prevention programs, experience with infectious disease outbreaks, and capacity for rapid response when an outbreak occurs. Additionally, cities benefit from ready access to healthcare facilities and medical professionals trained in many specialty areas. Nevertheless, low-income families sometimes have difficulty receiving adequate healthcare for infectious and other diseases due to the cost of medical services, limited health insurance options, unfamiliarity with health programs and services, and transportation and language barriers. This is especially true in developing nations, where many city residents may live in poverty.

Infectious disease control in cities will be even more important in the future as climate change results in the spread of insect-borne diseases due to warmer temperatures. Also, the rising occurrence of antibiotic-resistant bacteria will present a greater burden on healthcare systems to care for patients whose infections are difficult to control. Another issue already receiving considerable attention is the potential for international travelers to carry new and exotic diseases into the cities they visit. These and other issues will require enhanced funding for city healthcare programs and a high level of coordination among city, state, and federal infectious disease experts and agencies.

RECOMMENDATIONS FOR CITY DWELLERS

To avoid contracting an infectious disease, there are several common-sense steps that everyone should take, particularly city dwellers, who are at greater risk for exposure to infectious agents. These steps include the following:

- **Vaccinations.** Immunizations can dramatically reduce the risk of contracting many infectious diseases. Childhood vaccinations are especially important to keep children healthy and prevent infections that they may be exposed to in day care and at school. Additionally, adults need to be routinely vaccinated to prevent diseases such as tetanus and influenza, and older adults benefit from pneumococcal and shingles vaccinations. You can find CDC-recommended vaccinations by age group at www.cdc.gov/vaccines/vpd/vaccines-age.html.

- **Handwashing and good hygiene.** Practicing good hygiene is especially important. Wash your hands before eating and after using the toilet, and avoid touching your eyes, nose, and mouth with your hands. Do not share personal items, such as toothbrushes and razors, and avoid drinking from the same glass or using the same eating utensils as others.

- **Food preparation.** Keep food-preparation surfaces clean, cook foods to the recommended temperature, and wash fruits and vegetables thoroughly. Be sure to clean all cooking utensils carefully and to wash your hands before preparing meals. Leftovers should be promptly refrigerated.

- **Avoiding crowds.** To reduce your chance of catching a cold or the flu, avoid large crowds of people, particularly during the winter cold and flu season.

- **Staying home if you are sick.** To prevent your illness from spreading to others, stay home from work or school if you are sick. Staying home can also help you recover more quickly.

- **Practicing safe sex.** If you or your partner has a history of sexually transmitted disease or high-risk behavior, take appropriate precautions, including using condoms.

- **Travel precautions.** If traveling internationally, talk with your doctor about any special precautions, including getting vaccinations, avoiding certain regions, and drinking bottled water. Be especially diligent about good hygiene on cruise ships, where conditions are often conducive to the spread of *Norovirus* and other infectious diseases. Some medicines can provide short-term protection; for example, an antiparasitic medication may help you avoid contracting malaria. When preparing for a trip, you can find a list of CDC-recommended vaccinations at https://wwwnc.cdc.gov/travel/destinations/list.

If you are a patient in a hospital or other healthcare facility, you should be cautious about HAIs, which can quickly spread among patients and healthcare workers. Some steps to avoid HAIs include (1) talking with your doctor about your HAI concerns and asking what measures are being taken to protect you; (2) insisting that all the people you come into contact with wash their hands before touching you; (3) asking what types of tests will be performed to be sure that you are receiving the right antibiotic; (4) becoming familiar with the signs and symptoms of infection, such as redness, pain, drainage, or fever; (5) notifying your doctor immediately if you are having a problem with diarrhea; and (6) avoiding complications by getting vaccinated against the flu and other infections.

If you are feeling ill or have symptoms of an infection, seek medical attention right away. In particular, the Mayo Clinic recommends seeing your doctor if you experience any of the following:

- being bitten by an animal
- having trouble breathing
- coughing for more than a week
- having a severe headache with fever

- experiencing a rash or swelling
- having unexplained or prolonged fever
- experiencing sudden vision problems

When you have symptoms of the flu or other infections, a visit to your doctor's office can help prevent more serious complications and speed recovery.

CITY SPOTLIGHT: FREETOWN—CHECKING THE SPREAD OF A DEADLY VIRUS

When the Ebola epidemic overtook Freetown, city officials were slow to react, not understanding the seriousness of the outbreak and having limited resources to address the disease. With help from international aid agencies, the city defeated the virus, and in the process, health officials from around the world learned important lessons that can be applied to future disease outbreaks.

Ebola is a rare and severe viral infection that attacks the immune system, causing extreme fluid loss, and frequently death, within a week after initial symptoms appear. At the height of the 2014–2015 Ebola crisis in West Africa, Freetown, the capital city of Sierra Leone, was at the epicenter of the fight against this deadly virus. Because of its high population density, congested markets and streets, and limited healthcare services, Freetown and surrounding areas present ideal conditions for the spread of infectious diseases. Among the countries struck by the Ebola epidemic, Sierra Leone, with over 14,000 cases and nearly 4,000 deaths, was the hardest hit, and many of these deaths occurred in Freetown and its suburbs.

Freetown has a struggling economy and a limited infrastructure to support its population of over a million people. Despite the extreme poverty faced by many residents, especially those in the sprawling slum areas, people continue to come to the city from poor rural areas, seeking jobs and education. Founded by the British in 1787 as a home for freed slaves evacuated from Caribbean countries, the area has attracted a variety of people from various cultural and ethnic backgrounds, such that today, it has a very diverse population with varying cultural practices and beliefs. When the Ebola virus struck, Freetown was still recovering from a destructive civil war that left areas of the city and surrounding countryside in ruin. Poverty is rampant—one in five children die before age 5, more women die in childbirth than anywhere else in the world, and there are too few doctors, nurses, and healthcare facilities.

The city was initially slow to react to the epidemic, in part due to its limited resources, and also because the rapid spread of the disease caught many by surprise. When the magnitude of the epidemic became apparent, there were many more Ebola patients than hospital beds, and hospitals and health clinics were woefully understaffed. With help from the WHO and other international aid groups, a global contingent of doctors and nurses were flown in, existing healthcare facilities were upgraded, the ambulance fleet was expanded, and community-care centers were set up in neighborhoods with the greatest need. Because caregivers from outside the country are not always trusted, local residents were trained to assist with patient care and burials, and trusted entertainment personalities helped educate the public on early detection and treatment. These educational programs proved to be quite important because when the outbreak began, about a quarter of Freetown residents were reluctant to accept government intervention, believing that spiritual healers could treat Ebola better than medical professionals. (When families were suspected of hiding sick loved ones from government health workers, the government threatened them with jail time.)

Now that the Ebola epidemic has subsided and life in Freetown is getting back to normal, international health professionals are reflecting on lessons learned that can be applied to future epidemics of Ebola and other infectious agents. Perhaps the most important lesson is to understand the effect of local customs in spreading disease and to find solutions by working with the locals themselves. With Ebola, the best example of this involved the burials of Ebola victims, where ceremonial practices, including cleaning and dressing the body, sometimes delayed burial of the corpse for several days. Because the Ebola virus is often most infectious just before and after death, these hands-on burial practices, observed by many Freetown residents, were identified as one of the prime mechanisms for spreading the virus. Through coordination among health officials, religious leaders, and local chiefs, these unsanitary burial practices were replaced with burials performed almost immediately after death, where the body was first sealed in a body bag using sterile procedures. Family members were excluded from this process, although in deference to local customs, families were allowed to pray for the deceased, standing some distance away to avoid infection. Also, family members could leave money or jewelry to be placed in the body bag to help ensure their loved one's passage to the next world.

Many infectious disease experts believe that epidemics like the Ebola outbreak have less to do with the particular strain of virus and more to do with the presence of a weak healthcare system and inadequate city infrastructure. To fight future epidemics, cities need to be equipped with modern sewage systems, paved roads allowing healthcare workers better access to remote areas of the city, reliable electricity service, and a network of well-equipped and highly functioning hospitals. Of course, poverty also needs to be addressed, particularly in slum areas like those in Freetown, where up to three families may occupy the same household, sometimes living there in shifts due to limited space.

EXPERT COMMENTARY: "ONE HEALTH" POLICIES AND PRACTICES

Urbanization of infectious disease epidemics underlines the role of global interconnectedness as a driver of health.

Chadia Wannous, Coordinator

Toward a Safer World Network

Dr. Wannous is a public health professional specializing in emergency pre-paredness and response and in risk reduction of health threats. She has a par-ticular interest in risk drivers of diseases, including climate change, biodiversity, and urbanization. Dr. Wannous recently served as a senior advisor at the United Nations (UN) Office for Disaster Risk Reduction, coordinating imple-mentation of the health components of the Sendai Framework for Disaster Risk Reduction and managing the Science and Technology Secretariat. Prior to this, she was a senior policy advisor to the UN Secretary General Special Envoy on Ebola and to the UN System Influenza Coordinator. She is now coor-dinating the Towards a Safer World Network.

What do you see as the greatest issues regarding the implementation of "one health" policies and practices in urban areas, what are the major obstacles to addressing these issues, and what is your hope for the future?

One Health (OH) emerged in 2004 as a concept to foster interdisciplinary collaboration, as required to prevent and control zoonoses (diseases transmit-ted to humans from animals) among the human health, animal health, and wildlife sectors. It also extends to other sectors, such as trade, travel, and finance, and to other specialists like environmentalists, anthropologists, econ-omists, and sociologists. The OH approach has been promoted worldwide, given the high societal and economic risks of disease epidemics, to address issues at the interface between sectors beyond zoonoses (for example, food safety and security, antimicrobial resistance, and climate change). As the world becomes increasingly urbanized, effective prevention and control of diseases and implementation of the OH approach will center upon a better understanding of disease dynamics in urban settings.

Urbanization, fueled by global rural-to-urban migration fleeing economic or humanitarian hardships, is one of the main drivers of (1) emerging infec-tious diseases due to overcrowding, poor water and sanitation facilities, and impeachment of wildlife natural habitats; (2) noncommunicable diseases related to environmental determinants, such as injuries, indoor and outdoor air pollution, and climate change, causing dangerous stresses on public health and affecting lifestyle; (3) diseases related to poverty and inequities in access to affordable and quality healthcare; and (4) large cities in less-developed regions facing a higher risk of exposure to climate-related natural disasters, economic losses, and mortality than those in more developed regions.

Urbanization of infectious disease epidemics underlines the role of global interconnectedness as a driver of health. For example, outbreaks of Ebola virus disease were usually confined to small, remote areas in African countries prior to the 2014 epidemic in West Africa, when the disease reached the capital cities of Sierra Leone, Liberia, and Guinea. Interconnectedness in the cities exacerbates disease transmission risks within and across the borders of the three countries.

Urban and slum health should be considered a major development challenge and given adequate attention in ongoing health and climate initiatives if efforts to prevent and control disease and infection are to succeed. To do so, it is vital that we:

- Invest in and promote OH as a "whole of society and whole of government" approach to support early detection of disease threats at the source, leading to fewer outbreaks and effective response by establishing relationships and mechanisms for collaboration between health and nonhealth sectors to ensure preparedness capabilities are in place to detect, respond, and mitigate the effects of health threats across sectors and levels of governance.

- Develop a capable workforce across sectors that demonstrates the core competencies necessary to better understand future challenges posed by emerging threats and their risk drivers and to better manage and reduce health risks upstream.

- Invest in building healthy cities to put health high on the social, economic, and political agenda of city governments and to build strong public health at the local level. Creating heathier urban settings that support the health and well-being of the people, by enforcing building codes, promoting green and energy-efficient buildings, planting shade trees and forested green spaces, and other measures, will help communities become more resilient to the damaging impacts of climate change.

- Strengthen the overall health systems, including through better financing. This will enhance the performance of the system and also help reduce inequalities and accelerate achievement of universal health coverage.

- Build resilient and safe health infrastructure, such as the Climate Smart Healthcare and Green and Safe Health Infrastructure programs, to help countries address the burden of diseases, with potential benefits distributed among the sectors.

- Build an evidence base to improve our understanding of the drivers of disease emergence, many of which occur outside the health sector, including climate change, environmental degradation, and urbanization. This will help to systematically assess and integrate environmental dimensions along with human, agriculture, and animal health, targeting appropriate entry points through robust and risk-informed analysis and guiding risk-management and risk-reduction efforts.

- Mainstream disease prevention into national plans for climate change adaptation, biodiversity, sustainable development goals, the new urban agenda, and other relevant global frameworks to reduce health risks upstream and advance country progress, and advocate for combining resources and solutions among these frameworks for global and local public health.

As we transform our world, my hope that we do so by greater investment in sustainability through systems strengthening, research, and development and by adopting the OH approach to create synergies of strategies that address challenges faced due to health threats and urbanization.

Light Pollution

It is difficult to imagine a city without lighting. We depend on artificial lighting (light created by humans) for a wide range of nighttime activities that would otherwise be difficult, if not impossible. However, lighting can be a nuisance when it disturbs sleep or hinders stargazing. Furthermore, chronic exposure to artificial light has been associated with insomnia, depression, and even some serious physiological health concerns. When artificial light interferes with our lives and threatens our health, we refer to it as "light pollution."

Before cities became electrified and automobiles with headlights took over our streets, city residents could gaze on the sky above, making out several thousand stars, and even a few galaxies. However, those days are long gone, and today, with bright city lights, air pollution, and skyscrapers, we are fortunate if we can even catch a glimpse of the moon. Because of light pollution, only about one-third of people in the world can regularly see the Milky Way, and in the United States and other industrialized nations, just a few dozen stars can be seen by the residents of large metropolitan areas. Astronomers have complained about light pollution in cities for years, but the concept of excessive lighting as a form of pollution that can threaten public health is relatively new.

Urban light pollution is usually caused by street and highway lights, motor vehicle headlights, and outdoor lighting at homes and businesses. For example, a security light, neon sign, or streetlamp can cause light pollution if it is brighter than needed or unnecessarily spreads light over a broad area. In contrast with other forms of environmental pollution, light pollution problems can be easy to resolve, provided that everyone involved is willing to work together to find a satisfactory solution.

As an aid in describing light pollution problems and finding solutions, light pollution is often categorized as follows:

- **Sky glow**—a brightening of the sky over urban areas due to the collective contribution of light from thousands of streetlights and other sources. Sky glow allows many urban areas to be photographed at night by spacecraft.

- **Light trespass**—light that spreads into areas where it is neither needed nor wanted, such as a security light that shines into a neighbor's bedroom window.

- **Glare**—bright light that is distracting and can cause visual discomfort. Automobile headlights are often a source of bothersome glare.

The proliferation of trespassing and glaring lights in cities is symptomatic of another problem, which is that one-third to as much as three-fourths of the artificial light that we create at night is wasted. This means that a substantial amount of artificial light is unnecessary for our safety, navigation on sidewalks and streets, evening recreation, and commercial advertising. When city governments, residents, and businesses take actions to reduce wasted light, light pollution is reduced, and so are electric energy costs. In the United States, if all wasted light were eliminated, the cost savings would exceed $2 billion annually, with some estimates ranging as high as $10 billion. Furthermore, eliminating wasted light helps cut air pollution and fight climate change by reducing the amounts of carbon dioxide (CO_2) and other gases emitted into the atmosphere from fossil fuel–powered electric power plants.

In addition to affecting our health, wasting energy, and contributing to climate change, light pollution can be a problem for many species of birds that depend on stars for navigation and have their view of the sky obscured by bright city lights. Nocturnal animals that live in urban areas (e.g., bats, opossums, and raccoons) can also be disturbed by artificial lighting when it affects their circadian rhythms and interferes with their vision, foraging habits, and navigational instincts. Sometimes bright lights will attract moths and other insects, which in turn can entice hundreds of bats looking for a meal. Bats are unwelcome guests when they congregate near our homes and businesses because they are associated with human diseases, such as rabies and histoplasmosis (an infectious disease primarily affecting the lungs).

IMPACT ON URBAN HEALTH

Light pollution can affect our health in various ways. Exposure to bright light before bedtime can make us feel irritated and lead to insomnia, and repeated exposure over longer periods has been associated with depression, cardiovascular disease, and even cancer. Research studies indicate that exposure to bright light at night suppresses melatonin secretion and increases sleep onset latency, and the circadian misalignment associated with chronic nighttime bright light exposure may adversely affect psychological, cardiovascular, and metabolic functions. Even if the light is not bright, melatonin secretion and disruption of circadian rhythms can occur, especially for some light-emitting diode (LED), fluorescent, and metal halide lighting having shorter wavelengths that impart a blue-white color.

Some studies suggest that women exposed to artificial light during nightshift work may have an increased risk of breast cancer, perhaps due to changes in the levels of melatonin or other hormones. The American Cancer Society and Centers for Disease Control and Prevention (CDC) report that this is a fairly recent finding, and more research is needed to confirm it. On the other hand, the International Agency for Research on Cancer has taken a more aggressive stance, placing shiftwork involving circadian disruptions on their list of probable human carcinogens (Group 2A). A recent study of nearly 110,000 women performed by the Harvard T. H. Chan School of Public Health found that women living in areas with higher levels of outdoor light may be at higher risk for breast cancer, and this link was stronger among women who work night shifts.

Concern about LED street lighting have been raised by the American Medical Association (AMA), which has issued community guidance for reducing the harmful human and environmental effects of roadway lighting systems using LEDs. This type of high-intensity lighting consumes less energy than conventional lighting, resulting in lower reliance on fossil fuels to generate electricity, and about 10 percent of existing street lighting in the United States has already been converted to LED technology. However, according to the AMA, LED lighting emits large amounts of blue light that appears white to the naked eye and can cause a hazardous nighttime glare for drivers. Furthermore, because blue LED light suppresses melatonin at night, LED lighting has a fivefold-greater impact on disrupting circadian sleep rhythms compared with conventional street lighting. This can result in reduced sleep time, diminished sleep quality, impaired daytime functioning, and even obesity. The AMA guidelines recommend that communities use the lowest-intensity street lighting possible to minimize blue-rich light, shield the lights properly to minimize glare, and consider dimming the lights during off-peak periods.

Bright lighting on roadways can actually be hazardous to drivers because when our eyes adjust to the bright lights, we have difficulty seeing dimmer lights (e.g., when turning off a well-lit freeway onto a poorly lit local road). Similarly, when we leave a brightly lit gas station or roadside fast food restaurant, our eyes require some time to adjust to lower light levels, and during this adjustment period, we may not notice a deer crossing the road or a car stopped in front of us. While the quickest improvement in vision occurs during the first few minutes after leaving a brightly lit area, several hours are actually required for our eyes to adjust fully to darkness. Headlight glare from oncoming traffic can also be hazardous, causing us to momentarily take our eyes off the road in front of us. High-intensity headlights and fog lights are particularly distracting, especially if not aimed correctly. A recently study found that nearly half of the automobiles in the Unites States subject to annual safety inspections had one or two headlights that were improperly aimed.

WHAT CITIES ARE DOING ABOUT LIGHT POLLUTION

Many cities have enacted light-pollution guidelines for public facilities and also regulations for privately owned facilities, often incorporated into city zoning codes. A common objective is simply to eliminate all lighting that is unnecessary for safety. This may include landscape lighting, excessive street lighting, and indoor lights after business hours. (Businesses often cooperate in reducing unnecessary lighting because doing so reduces their electricity bills.) Dusk-to-dawn sensors are frequently used to ensure that outdoor lights are off during daylight hours, as are timers that turn lights on and off at specific times of the day. Motion sensors, common in newer buildings, turn off lights when a room is unoccupied.

In addition to eliminating unnecessary lighting, other approaches specified by cities to reduce light pollution include:

- Replacing needlessly bright lights with lower-intensity lighting, resulting not only in less light pollution, but also lower electricity bills and less air pollution from fossil fuel–powered electric power plants.

- Orienting light in the direction that does the most good and adding shielding to prevent light from spreading to areas where it is not needed.

(When light fixtures are properly aimed, lower-wattage light bulbs can often be used.)

- Equipping windows with awnings, blinds, or shades (including automatic shades) to prevent indoor light from spreading outside during evening hours.
- Regulating the size of outdoor commercial signs and locating other outdoor lighting away from residential buildings, unless needed for security.

Security lights are often located over entry doors or in dark areas where vandalism and other mischief may occur. They can be bright and intrusive, however, and reducing light pollution from this type of lighting is sometimes challenging because it is not always possible to position these lights where they are not visible from residential property or the street. Fortunately, there are several options that can be quite effective in reducing the impact of security lighting on neighboring properties and are commonly employed through urban areas, including equipping outdoor light fixtures with motion detection switches that turn the light on when someone is nearby and turn it off when the person leaves the area, installing light fixture shielding, and using a spotlight in place of a floodlight. (Spotlights narrowly focus light rather than allowing it to spread over a wide area.)

One effective way to identify unnecessary lighting is to conduct an energy audit, which is an investigation into how energy is used and whether any is wasted. When performed by city governments at public facilities, lighting is often identified as a significant source of wasted energy. For example, many cities have realized substantial electricity cost savings simply by turning off parking lot and office lights during overnight periods, when they are not needed, and by removing light bulbs from vending machines. Eliminating excessive roadway lighting has also achieved major reductions in energy costs—and light pollution—in some cities.

Some cities and states have implemented measures to specifically address concerns about bright highways, such as reducing bright lighting and replacing roadway lights with small headlight reflectors positioned between lanes. Reflectors can be quite effective in defining roadway lanes without exposing drivers to excessive light. Additionally, a number of states have enacted laws to reduce light pollution, often applying to state-owned facilities and roadways where public funds are used. While each state's laws are unique, many of these laws share the following features:

- Requiring shields on light fixtures that direct the light downward and allow the use of lower-wattage bulbs
- Using low-glare or low-wattage lights where shielding is not feasible, or in addition to shielding
- Illuminating areas with only as much light as is necessary and eliminating light trespass
- Limiting the amount of time that lighting is used, switching off lighting after a certain hour (e.g., midnight), and installing automatic on/off switches

Several state laws are designed to preserve the natural night environment or the rural character of an area, and some laws are intended to minimize the effect of beachfront lighting on birds and marine life (e.g., protecting nesting and hatching sea turtles from artificial light). Other laws are aimed at reducing unnecessary lighting around military bases and encouraging options to installing new roadway lighting, such as reducing the speed limit, painting lines on road surfaces, and relying on headlight reflectors and informational signs. Construction and emergency lighting is often exempt from state light pollution regulations.

RECOMMENDATIONS FOR CITY DWELLERS

Try to avoid brightly lit surroundings at night, especially close to bedtime, and resist watching television or checking the computer later in the evening. To get a good night's rest and avoid disrupting your circadian rhythms, sleep in a dark bedroom and be sure to turn off all electronic devices while sleeping. For people who often wake up during the night, resist checking cell-phone messages or turning on a bright bathroom light. Research indicates that a dim red light in the bathroom provides sufficient light in the middle of the night, and red light suppresses melatonin production to a lesser degree than other colors. Some computer and cell-phone screens have an evening setting that reduces the blue light associated with melatonin suppression and shifting circadian rhythms.

Taking melatonin tablets before bedtime is thought to be helpful in regulating sleep-wake cycles and circadian rhythms. However, studies show mixed results, and because of potential side effects, interactions with medications, and special concerns for young people, individuals should consult a medical professional before taking melatonin or giving it to children.

Some potential side effects associated with melatonin include headaches, nausea, grogginess the next day, fluctuations in hormone levels, and vivid dreams and nightmares. The National Center for Complementary and Integrative Health reports that "researchers have conducted many studies on whether melatonin supplements may help people with various sleep disorders. However, important questions remain about its usefulness, how much to take, when to take it, and its long-term safety. . . . Melatonin supplements appear to be safe when used short-term; less is known about long-term safety."

Homeowners should consider taking an evening stroll around their property to investigate any sources of unnecessary light and see what can be done about it. If the light originates on someone else's property, the property owner may be willing to (1) remove unnecessary lights or switch them off at bedtime; (2) use low-wattage bulbs or spotlights; (3) install motion-detecting switches so that the light turns on only if a person or animal is nearby; and (4) employ shielding or aim the light away from other properties. Another option is to block light from entering windows by using shades, blinds, or awnings.

To avoid being distracted by vehicle headlight glare, drivers can try looking down and away while the vehicle passes, focusing on the white line on the passenger's side of the road. Using peripheral vision, the driver will still be able to see the vehicle, but its bight headlights will be less distracting. Keeping the front windshield clean (both inside and outside) can also be helpful because dirt and grime on the windshield can refract oncoming headlights, making the glare even worse. To reduce the headlight glare from behind, drivers should use the night setting on the rear-view mirror, which changes the angle of the mirror's reflective surface, making the headlights appear less intense. (Some automobiles now come equipped with self-dimming mirrors.)

Antiglare eyeglass coating can help reduce headlight glare. However, eye care professionals warn against wearing sunglasses at night because they can make night vision worse by restricting the light entering the eyes. Furthermore, as the eyes become accustomed to the sunglasses, they may offer reduced protection during daylight hours. Routine vision examinations are important, especially as we grow older and our eyes become more sensitive to light. Older adults are more prone to cataracts, which make headlight glare even worse, and older eyes take longer to readjust to changing lighting conditions. The eyes of a 55-year-old may take eight times longer to recover from glare than those of a 16-year-old, a statistic that will become a more serious concern for many nations as their population ages. The best option to cope with headlight glare may simply be to avoid driving at night.

As a courtesy to other drivers during nighttime driving, keep your automobile headlights clean (a dirty headlight may cause more glare for an approaching car) and ensure that the headlights are properly aimed as part of routine maintenance at an automobile dealer or repair shop. During foggy conditions, avoid using the high-beam headlights, and when the fog clears, be sure to turn off fog lamps if the car is equipped with them. Never use high beams in urban areas and when you can see oncoming traffic.

Noise Pollution

When asked what one word comes to mind to describe the city environment, people often say "noise." In the city, noise is all around us—traffic congestion along busy thoroughfares, the construction of new buildings, subway trains screeching to a halt, and the chatter of patrons in coffee shops and cafés are all familiar sounds of the city. A little background noise is not a problem for most of us, but when the mixture of sounds becomes too loud for too long, our health can suffer.

One way to learn about the noise problems in a city is by scanning the newspapers. For example, the local news section of *The New York Times* recently reported citizen complaints about deafening subway trains, construction clamor, excessive noise from leaf blowers, barking dogs, loud parties next door, and a rowdy sidewalk café. Residents even complained about ice cream truck jingles playing nonstop on loudspeakers all day long. It is no wonder that soundproofing contractors in New York City and other metropolitan areas are busier than ever addressing noise complaints. Some of these gripes may seem trivial, but to the person wanting a quiet place to read a book or fall asleep, almost any unwanted sound can be annoying.

When the majority of the world's population lived in small towns, villages, and farming communities, noise was seldom a problem. However, as cities expanded and population densities increased, people found themselves living in close proximity to commercial and industrial areas and to each other, and noise complaints became more commonplace. To address these concerns, governments enacted laws aimed at reducing noise to acceptable levels, although what constitutes an acceptable level has always been an issue. Most jurisdictions agree that noise loud enough to damage hearing should be prevented, but what about noises that are annoying or intrusive, but do not cause permanent hearing loss? The level of noise control in cities is often a compromise between the right of residents to live in a reasonably quiet environment and the right of companies to conduct business. Some noises just have to be accepted as part of city life, such as automobiles on a busy street or neighbors having an occasional party.

Noise is a global issue, and while no two cities have exactly the same noise problems, the major source of noise in almost every large urban area is traffic. It is difficult to know just how many people living in cities are subjected to excessive noise from traffic and other sources. However, the World Health Organization (WHO) estimates that about 40 percent of the European population is exposed to significant road traffic noise, and 20 percent is affected by nighttime noise from various sources. Additionally, according to the WHO, over 1 billion teenagers and young adults (ages 12–35) worldwide are at risk of hearing loss resulting from exposure to noise in recreational settings, such as use of personal audio devices at high volumes and for prolonged periods of time and regular attendance at concerts, nightclubs, bars, and sporting events. In the United States, the Centers for Disease Control and Prevention (CDC) reports that about 17 percent of adults have suffered permanent hearing damage due to excessive exposure to noise.

IMPACT ON URBAN HEALTH

City noises affect our health in two ways. First, loud, continuous noise can damage our hearing, particularly at higher frequencies. Second, incessant noise can take a psychological toll by interfering with thoughts and emotions, sometimes making us feel angry or apathetic. And as our mental stress builds up, we may experience sleepless nights, poor work and school performance, interference with speech, elevated blood pressure, and stress-related illnesses. Because we cannot see, taste, smell, or touch noise pollution, as we can with other forms of urban pollution, we usually do not consider noise a direct threat to our health. However, when noise diminishes our ability to hear and adds to our daily stress level, our health and well-being can be seriously threatened.

Loud noise can also be an occupation hazard in the workplace. The U.S. Occupational Safety and Health Administration (OSHA) has established rules to protect the hearing of workers from elevated noise levels while on the job, and most companies having noisy operations try to moderate loud noises and ensure their workers wear ear protection. Even so, American companies spend more than $200 million annually on workers' compensation for hearing loss disabilities and pay over $1 million in penalties. OSHA estimates that 22 million workers are exposed to potentially harmful noise every year.

How loud is too loud? Scientific instruments that measure sound levels use a unit of measure called the "decibel (dB)"—the higher the dB, the louder the sound. Because dBs are measured using a logarithmic scale, for every 10-dB increase in noise, the perceived loudness doubles. The effects of different dB levels are listed here:

- 20 dB—the sound level is just barely audible
- 30 dB—a very quiet room
- 50–60 dB—a comfortable level of hearing
- 80 dB—sounds loud enough to interfere with conversation
- 85 dB—the sound level where hearing damage may occur after 8 hours of exposure
- 90–100 dB—unprotected exposure should be limited to no more than 15 minutes
- Over 100 dB—regular exposure above this sound level risks permanent hearing loss
- 125 dB—generally considered the threshold of pain for loud sounds

Many activities that we take for granted, such as attending a concert, operating a power saw, and firing a shotgun, can permanently reduce our ability to hear sounds over a range of frequencies. Even riding a motorcycle, operating a lawnmower, and running a food blender can harm your hearing if the noise level is high enough or continues over an extended period. According to the CDC, listening to a deafening rock concert for as little as two minutes can permanently damage your hearing. Table 14 lists the noise levels associated with some common urban sounds.

Sometimes noise levels are reported as dB(A), which is the standard dB scale adjusted to take into account how sensitive the human ear is to certain frequencies of sound, and which is believed to correlate better with the risk of noise-induced hearing loss. The WHO recommends less than 30 dB(A) of noise for good-quality sleep, and less than 35 dB(A) for good teaching and learning conditions in the classroom. Another adjustment,

Table 14   Noise Levels Associated with Some Common Urban Sounds

Sound	Typical Noise Level (dB)
Normal breathing	10
Rustling leaves	20
Whisper	30
Refrigerator humming	40
Normal conversation	50–60
Vacuum cleaner, hair dryer	70
Dishwasher	75
Washing machine	78
Average city traffic	80
Diesel truck	84
Lawnmower, food blender	85–90
Subway, motorcycle	88
Garbage truck, cement mixer	100
Jet flyover	103
Chainsaw, pneumatic drill, jackhammer	110
Stereo (100 watts)	110–125
Thunderclap	120
Rock concert	110–140
Shotgun, jet takeoff	130
Jet engine	140

Source: National Institute on Deafness and Other Communication Disorders.

known as the "dB(C) scale," is sometimes used to characterize high sound levels, such as nearby gunfire.

A condition known as "noise-induced hearing loss (NIHL)" is the most common effect of living and working in a noisy environment. NIHL is a very common health condition in the United States and throughout the

Table 15   U.S. Adults Having Disabling Hearing Loss

Age Range	Percentage with Hearing Loss
45–54	2
55–64	8.5
65–74	25
75 and older	50

Source: National Institute on Deafness and Other Communication Disorders.

developed world, and unfortunately, it is ordinarily irreversible. Working in a noisy factory can cause NIHL, but so can attending a loud concert or even using a noisy leaf blower. Typically, the louder the sound and the longer the exposure, the greater the likelihood of permanent hearing loss is. Among U.S. adults age 20–69, about 40 million suffer from NIHL. Because half of these adults do not have noisy jobs, their hearing loss must be associated with noise exposure elsewhere in the community (e.g., at school or home). Of those U.S. adults who think their hearing is good to excellent, about 25 percent actually have some degree of hearing damage. Table 15 lists the percentage of U.S. adults having disabling hearing loss.

Hearing loss often becomes more severe as we get older. The National Institute on Deafness and Other Communication Disorders reports that disabling hearing loss (35 dB or more in the better ear, the level at which adults generally benefit from hearing aids) affects one-quarter of Americans between the ages of 65 and 74 and half of people over 75. Aging-related hearing loss, known as "presbycusis," is a concern for older adults living in the city because they may have difficulty hearing a smoke or fire alarm, and their hearing loss can lead to feelings of isolation. Older adults are also prone to suffer more from sleep disruption and mental stress caused by noise. High blood pressure, diabetes, and other medical conditions common in older adults can contribute to hearing loss, as can certain medications, such as chemotherapy drugs. Typically, hearing loss in older adults is associated with both presbycusis and NIHL.

Children can also suffer from hearing loss, and research indicates that chronic exposure to noise can harm a child's cognitive performance, motivation, and overall well-being. Additionally, because children spend more time in bed than adults, their sleep can be more affected by nighttime noise. Low-income families represent another population group affected by noise. These families often cannot afford to live in quiet suburbs, and consequently, they may be disproportionately exposed to city noise, resulting in increased expenses for medical care and medications and lower performance at work and school. Because of these disproportionate affects, the WHO suggests that noise pollution may have the effect of increasing the income gap between rich and poor.

Many people throughout the world, including over 50 million Americans, also suffer from tinnitus, a ringing or buzzing in the ears that is most often caused by prolonged exposure to loud noise. (It can also be caused by the buildup of earwax, certain health conditions and illnesses, and some drugs.) Tinnitus can disrupt sleep and concentration, reduce alertness, and increase fatigue, and according to the American Tinnitus Association, half or more of patients with severe tinnitus experience depression, anxiety, or some other behavioral disorder. Also, most people with tinnitus have some level of hearing loss. The likelihood of developing tinnitus increases with age, and it is estimated that roughly 30 percent of older adults (over age 60) experience tinnitus symptoms. Other groups at high risk for developing tinnitus are active military personnel and veterans, people working in loud workplace environments, musicians and music lovers, motor sports fans, and hunters. Males tend to get tinnitus more than females, perhaps because they have noisier jobs and participate in more hearing-risk behaviors like hunting. For unknown reasons, white, non-Hispanic people suffer more from tinnitus than other racial and ethnic groups. In the United States, about 2 million people have tinnitus severe enough to be debilitating

WHAT CITIES ARE DOING ABOUT NOISE POLLUTION

Noise regulations are typically enacted at all levels of government, although local ordinances are usually the most effective for addressing the large variety of noises found in urban areas. In the United States, the federal government regulates only certain specific sources of noise, such as aircraft and airports, federally funded highway and housing projects, interstate motor carriers and railroads, medium- and heavy-duty trucks, motorcycles and mopeds, air compressors and other types of equipment, human activities in national parks and other federal lands, and occupation exposure to dangerous sounds. The enactment of ordinances to limit other sources of sounds, including many noises common to the urban environment, is left to state and local governments.

Some sound ordinances restrict sounds above a certain dB level, whereas others are more subjective, such as restrictions on sounds loud enough to be considered a nuisance. Ordinances may be more stringent during the evening or overnight hours when most people are sleeping, and they may limit certain activities to specified periods, such as restricting outdoor construction to weekdays and business hours. City officials typically do not go out looking for noise ordinance violations but instead react to complaints, usually made to the police department. Depending on the circumstances (e.g., time of day, noise level, and type of activity), a police officer may request that the noise level be lowered or some corrective action taken. For repeated complaints, a fine might be assessed or a business permit revoked. Unfortunately, the enforcement of noise ordinances can be highly variable and subjective, and many city governments have insufficient personnel and equipment to monitor compliance with the law.

Local zoning and land-use policies can help keep noisy delivery vehicles, mechanical equipment (e.g., rooftop ventilation systems), restaurants, and bars away from residential areas. Additionally, cities can restrict certain activities, such as truck deliveries and outdoor music, to specific times of the day, and quiet zones can be established near hospitals, schools, and other noise-sensitive establishments. To further limit the sound entering residences, local building codes can require sound-reducing construction techniques (e.g., thick walls incorporating acoustical insulation), and for existing residential construction, cities can subsidize improvements such as double-pane windows that also help reduce energy losses. These same techniques also can be required for noisy restaurants and bars to keep noise inside the building. Cities and counties in California are required to adopt a general plan for future development that includes provisions for addressing major noise sources, establishing noise contours for the community, protecting sensitive locations like hospitals, and developing methods to protect residents from excess noise.

The most common source of urban noise is traffic on city roads and on freeways passing through town, and unfortunately, the options for reducing this type of noise are limited. However, federal regulations limit truck engine noise, and automobiles have become quieter thanks to state and local statutes requiring mufflers to be in good working order and in constant operation. These statutes often prohibit muffler bypasses and other modifications that can make engines sound louder. Some states even require automobile exhaust noise to be below a specified dB level when measured next to or near the vehicle. Freeway and major thoroughfare noise can be reduced by as much as 50 percent by constructing sound barrier walls or berms and by planting dense vegetation, and alternative truck routes can keep large trucks away from congested areas. (The sound energy from a heavy truck can be over 20 times greater than a personal automobile.) Some cities address both the noise and air pollution from buses and sanitation trucks by using electric and hybrid vehicles, synchronizing traffic lights to minimize stops and starts at intersections, and limiting vehicle speed through urban areas.

Even with all of these noise reduction measures in place, urban residents can suffer from unwanted noise associated with their jobs. While at work, reducing sounds by even a few dBs can help protect hearing, while improving communication with fellow workers and reducing workday stress. Most companies are conscientious about protecting worker hearing, and some even provide quiet rooms, where workers can seek relief from loud and annoying workday noise. To reduce occupational sound levels, employers commonly take the following steps:

- Requiring workers to wear hearing-protective devices, including earmuffs and earplugs
- Implementing engineering controls, such as using low-noise tools and machinery, and placing a sound barrier between the noise source and the employee
- Applying administrative controls, including operating noisy equipment during shifts where fewer people are exposed, limiting the amount of time that workers are exposed to loud sounds, and locating workstations farther from noisy equipment
- Providing a hearing-conservation program, where (1) noise levels are monitored and hearing tests are routinely performed; (2) follow-up procedures are implemented if hearing loss is detected; (3) hearing protection equipment is selected based on individual needs; and (4) training is provided on avoiding excessive noise and using protective equipment correctly

A type of noise sometimes encountered in urban environments and on the job involves very low-frequency sounds and vibrations emanating from rotating industrial and construction equipment, large air conditioning systems, entertainment venues, and "boom cars" equipped with amplified music systems that are popular with some young people. (The sound levels in some boom cars can reach 150 dB and be heard from a long distance away.) Low-frequency sounds are often subaudible (i.e., their frequency is too low to be detected by the human ear) and difficult to measure, although we may be able to feel the vibration. One approach used to limit low-frequency sounds is to enact a local ordinance stating that no person should permit any sound emanating from their property or vehicle that can be clearly heard or felt within a specified distance (e.g., 50 feet, or 15 meters) of their property line or vehicle.

RECOMMENDATIONS FOR CITY DWELLERS

There are several steps that individuals living in the city can take to prevent hearing loss. The most important is simply limiting exposure to loud noise—walking away from the noise, lowering the volume, or wearing hearing protection, such as earplugs or earmuffs. And people need to be careful wearing headphones and earbuds—there is increasing evidence they can cause hearing loss if the volume is too loud. Parents can help their children avoid hearing loss by turning the volume down on televisions and music players and requiring ear protection while working outside, such as when using a lawn mower or leaf blower. To block out unwanted sounds, some people even wear earmuffs or headphones while walking on busy city streets or riding the subway.

It is important to pay attention to the intensity of sounds because when sound waves are strong enough to damage the sensory hair cells in the ear, the hair cells do not grow back or repair themselves, resulting in permanently diminished hearing. To determine if someone has significant hearing loss, a simple screening test can often be administered by a primary care physician, and sometimes schools and employers also offer screening tests. More detailed audiometric testing (hearing tests) can be performed by an audiologist, who specializes in identifying and measuring the types and degrees of hearing loss, or an otolaryngologist, who is a physician specializing in the diagnosis and treatment of diseases of the ear, nose, throat, and neck. Hearing aid specialists also test hearing, recommend types of hearing aids, and provide hearing aid fitting and testing services for their clients.

The opposite of noise is quiet, and there is an increasing body of knowledge suggesting that quiet itself can be highly beneficial to good health.

Quiet environments can be relaxing, thereby reducing stress and improving the ability to concentrate and perform complex tasks. Consumer demand has increased for quiet appliances in the home, and manufacturers have responded with dishwashers, refrigerators, and other home products so quiet that you hardly know they are operating. Additionally, new apartments and condominiums in urban areas often have bedrooms located at the back of the building, away from the noisy street in front. City residents also seek quiet in public areas such as libraries and parks. An early-morning stroll through a quiet neighborhood park may be all that is needed to start the day on a positive note.

Not all noise is bad. In fact, a little background noise—people talking at a sidewalk café, a delivery truck making its rounds, or a dog barking in the distance—reminds us that we are part of a community and helps provide social connectedness. Natural sounds in the city, like chirping birds and the rustling of leaves on a breezy day, are also pleasant to the ear. People take comfort in these muted urban sounds that make up the soundscape of the city. However, once the noise goes above about 50 dB, we start to become more aware of our noisy city surroundings and need to be prepared to protect our hearing if the sound level increases.

EXPERT COMMENTARY: ADDRESSING NOISE POLLUTION

My hope for the future is that education about noise, improved ease of reporting noise, and society's understanding of access to quiet as a human right will accelerate.

Jeanine Botta, Consultant

The Right to Quiet Society for Soundscape Awareness and Protection

Jeanine Botta is an activist and blogger specializing in vehicle noise and soundscape education. Working with the Right to Quiet Society for Soundscape Awareness and Protection, a Canadian nonprofit with global membership, she provides guidance about addressing various noise issues and education about the health benefits of access to quiet.

What do you see as the greatest issues regarding noise in urban areas, what are the major obstacles to addressing the issues, and what is your hope for the future?

Common issues involving noise in urban areas are indoor and outdoor residential sounds affecting neighbors, sounds emanating from entertainment venues, transportation sounds, and sounds from construction projects. Each of these categories has at least several subcategories, and some intersect with suburban issues, such as lawn maintenance noise. Transportation sounds include noise from traffic, rail and subway trains, and airplanes and helicopters, which are used as a means of transportation by the affluent and for urban tourism and tourism in national parks. Aircraft noise involving airline flight paths over residences also occurs in urban and suburban areas. It may not be possible to say which noise issue has the greatest impact because noise-complaint statistics are not reliable.

Many individuals who are affected by noise do not complain for several reasons, including fear of retaliation and belief that complaints will not be taken seriously. Individuals who complain multiple times, intending to quantify the problem, are dismissed as serial complainers rather than being perceived as activists or citizen scientists. Some elected leaders are sympathetic to one type of noise and dismissive of others, partly because of their subjective experiences and beliefs. All of these scenarios serve as obstacles to addressing noise, resulting in seemingly low complaint levels, and giving elected leaders the impression that few constituents are affected by noise.

There is growing interest in technology, as tech start-ups install audio sensors in urban locations as a means of mapping noise pollution. And smartphone apps enable everyone to contribute to noise maps, allowing anyone to take part in citizen science, capturing quiet green spaces and reporting noisy streets. We can also submit sound levels and subjective data from restaurants and bars to identify and map quiet and noisy venues. But sound sensors will ultimately need to be placed in many more locations to capture reliable information beyond a few areas, and even the most robust noise data will not guarantee effective enforcement.

My hope for the future is that education about noise, improved ease of reporting noise, and society's understanding of access to quiet as a human right will accelerate. Sound education modules and student sound walks have been introduced in some cities. Technology to automate enforcement of noise ordinances is being used to address traffic noise outside of North America. And retailers now offer quiet hours for sound sensitive shoppers, including people with autism.

Those of us whose work has led to these and other improvements need to leave our silos, increase our knowledge, integrate our efforts, take great care not to fall victim to battle fatigue, refuse to settle, and support and mentor a new generation that seems to have a great interest in sound.

Odor Pollution

If it smells bad, it must be bad for you. That is what many people believe about odors, but this is not always the case. Countless substances having a pungent smell are harmless, while other odorless substances may cause serious health problems. Nevertheless, no one likes being around something that smells bad. Historically, odor complaints represent a large fraction of the citizen complaints made to city health departments and environmental agencies.

Many odors are associated with human activities, such as collecting garbage, making compost, or operating diesel-fueled vehicles. Other odors emanate from industrial operations, including oil refineries, landfills, paper mills, and wastewater treatment plants. Concentrated animal-feeding operations (agricultural operations where animals are confined to a lot or facility) can also be sources of offensive odors. Natural sources of odors include hydrogen sulfide gas emitted during a volcanic eruption, smoke from a forest fire, and moist soil following rain.

Among the five senses, our ability to smell is the most complex. Humans can distinguish over 10,000 different odors, some of which are perceived as pleasant and others the opposite. Pleasant odors help us enjoy a delicious meal at our favorite restaurant or a walk through the woods on a cool spring morning, while unpleasant odors can sometimes indicate a hazard, such as a gas leak. Odors are important in stimulating appetite and bringing to memory important events in our past, but having to live with unpleasant odors in a community can diminish the quality of life and sense of well-being. While humans are excellent in distinguishing odors, it is interesting that we almost always have great difficulty describing them in words.

There are four characteristics that determine our perception of odor—how strong the odor is and whether it is pleasant or unpleasant. The first characteristic is "detectability," which refers to the minimum concentration of a substance in the air that we can smell. (Our noses cannot detect concentrations lower than this minimum level.) Because detectability varies from person to person, someone may be able to detect a faint odor that another person misses. Nevertheless, the ability to detect odors is similar for most people.

The second characteristic of odor is "intensity," which refers to whether the odor is perceived as strong or weak. Intensity increases with the concentration of the substance in the air.

The third characteristic is "character," which is what the odor smells like or reminds us of. Odors often have a smell described as fishy, nutty, or rancid, or suggestive of ammonia, creosote, hay, sewer gas, or turpentine. Sometimes we can recognize specific substances or their sources from their smell.

The fourth characteristic of odor is "hedonic tone," which represents subjective judgment about whether an odor is pleasant or unpleasant. (The word "hedonic" is derived from the Greek word "hedone," which means pleasure.) A variety of factors influence hedonic tone, including the odor's intensity, character, duration, and frequency of occurrence. Location and time of day can also be factors. For example, freshly baked bread may smell wonderful during an early-morning visit to a local bakery, but if you live in an apartment above the bakery and are trying to fall asleep at night, the odor could be quite annoying. Table 16 illustrates our perception of different types of odors as pleasant or offensive.

In the field of odor science, two important concepts to understand are (1) the "detection threshold," which is the lowest concentration of an odor that is perceivable by the human sense of smell; and (2) the "recognition threshold," which is the lowest concentration where the odor can be identified. If the concentration is above the detection threshold but below the recognition threshold, a person may be able to detect the presence of an odor but not be able to identify it. Another concept is "olfactory fatigue," the temporary inability to distinguish an odor, which may occur when someone is exposed to an odor for a prolonged period of time. For example, dairy workers routinely exposed to the smell of manure may become unaware of the odor while performing their daily duties. A similar concept, "odor adaption," occurs when someone becomes accustomed to an odor, effectively increasing the detection threshold.

Table 16   How We Perceive Different Odors

Human Perception	Odor Characterization	Examples
Not unpleasant	Floral, herbal, pine, and minty smells	Alcohols
		Perfume
		Fresh-cut grass or hay
		Coffee roasting
		Bakery
		Winery
Unpleasant	Fishy, earthy, musty, musky, stale, soapy, chemical, and medicinal smells	Sewage treatment
		Cattle operation
		Diesel exhaust
		Asphalt plant
		Burned food
		Tobacco smoke
		Some local industries
Offensive	Pungent, rancid, and fecal smells	Landfill garbage
		Hog and poultry operations
		Decaying compost
		Grease-trap odor
		Waste burning (other than wood)
		Improperly operated septic system
Highly offensive	Putrid, rotten, and marshy smells	Untreated sewage
		Decaying animals
		Animal slaughterhouse
		Rotten grease
		Hydrogen sulfide (e.g., from paper mills, landfills, or volcanos)
		Mercaptans (added to natural gas to make leaks easier to detect)

Source: U.S. Agency for Toxic Substances and Disease Registry.

IMPACT ON URBAN HEALTH

Although odors are usually harmless, there are far more complaints about them than other air pollutants, and sometimes people attribute their illness symptoms to odors even though there is no toxicological evidence to back up such claims. On the other hand, some odors do cause adverse health reactions or indicate the presence of other air pollutants that may be harmful. Because hazardous chemicals can sometimes be smelled before their concentrations build up to harmful levels, these odors can act as a warning signal to contain the chemical or evacuate the area.

Our understanding of how people respond to odors is very complex because of a variety of factors that may vary by individual, including genetics, medical history, lifestyle, and personal preferences for liking or disliking certain odors. People with mental depression and certain medical conditions, such as asthma, chronic obstructive pulmonary disease (COPD), frequent headaches and migraines, and seizures, may be more sensitive to odors, and tobacco smoking and alcohol abuse may also increase sensitivity. Women tend to be more symptomatic from odor exposure than men, perhaps because women generally have a keener sense of smell. The ability to smell decreases with age, and up to one-third of older adults have lost the ability to detect the mercaptan added to natural gas to make it easier to detect gas leaks (as discussed later in this entry).

Some odors can cause adverse health experiences, depending on the substance causing the odor, the concentration in the air, how long and often exposure occurs, and a person's age, general health condition, and sensitivity to the substance. Examples of odor symptoms are headaches and dizziness, nasal congestion, sore throat, coughing and wheezing, chest tightness, shortness of breath, heart palpitations, nausea, drowsiness, and irritation of the eye, nose, and throat. Strong odors can interfere with outdoor activities and sleep, and if the odor is associated with a toxic chemical, serious health episodes may occur. In some cases, the substance causing an odor can worsen asthma, COPD, and emphysema. In general, as odor concentrations increase, the symptoms will worsen, and a greater number of people will have symptoms.

Children may be more sensitive to odors, in part because they have a faster breathing rate and play close to the ground, where odors heavier than air may accumulate. Odors also represent a special concern for older adults, who may be less sensitive to some odors due to existing illnesses and compromised immune systems. Because the sense of smell tends to decrease with age, an older adult may have difficulty detecting an odor that others find objectionable, with the result that the older adult remains exposed for a longer period of time. Pregnant women may also exhibit a greater sensitivity to odors.

Some hazardous substances have no odor, making detection difficult. For example, natural gas (methane), which is widely used in the United States for heating and cooking, is odorless, colorless, and tasteless, making leak detection difficult. This is a problem because if a natural gas leak occurs in a furnace or gas range and gas concentrations build up, an explosion and fire can occur. To make natural gas leaks easier to detect, a harmless but smelly substance called "mercaptan" (also known as "methyl mercaptan" and "methanethiol") is routinely added to the gas, giving the mixture an odor similar to rotten eggs.

Carbon monoxide (CO) is another example of a substance that has no detectible odor. CO occurs when fuels are combusted in engines, stoves, lanterns, grills, fireplaces, gas ranges, and furnaces. If the fuels are used in an enclosed area with poor ventilation, the CO can increase to dangerous levels, resulting in CO poisoning that can kill you. Common symptoms of CO poisoning include headache, dizziness, vomiting, chest pain, and confusion, and sometimes CO symptoms are described as flulike. People who are asleep or drunk can die from CO poisoning before knowing they have symptoms. According to the Centers for Disease Control and Prevention (CDC), over 400 Americans die each year from accidental CO poisoning (excluding fires), and more than 20,000 visit emergency rooms.

WHAT CITIES ARE DOING ABOUT ODOR POLLUTION

Odor complaints are often difficult for city health departments and environmental agencies to address because what is offensive to one person may not be to another. For example, you may love the smell of baked lasagna from an Italian restaurant down the street, but your neighbor, who dislikes Italian food, may find it offensive. Because our perception of odor is subjective, and because people have different sensitivities to different odors, arriving at a solution that satisfies everyone can be tricky.

If the odor is an ongoing problem that has the potential to affect health or quality of life, local officials may have the authority under zoning, nuisance, or other city ordinances to require the facility causing the odor to modify its operations or take other actions to reduce the odor. Also, zoning restrictions can sometimes prevent odor-creating factories or commercial operations from building or expanding near residential neighborhoods. Another approach is to require the facility to reduce or cease operation during times of the day or week when the odors are most bothersome, or during periods when local meteorology causes odors to build up to unacceptable levels (e.g., during an air pollution inversion). Faced with ongoing odor problems, some communities have developed educational materials for healthcare providers and the public on recognizing, reporting, and avoiding offensive odors.

The best approach to odor control is simply to prevent odors from being generated in the first place. For example, an industrial facility may be able to modify its operations by using chemicals and other raw materials that do not cause odors. When this is not possible, other options include (1) diluting the odorous gases with clean air; (2) dispersing the gases with a tall smokestack; (3) capturing and removing the gases using filtering or scrubbing technologies; (4) destroying the gases by incinerating them with afterburners or other combustion technologies; and (5) masking or neutralizing the odors by adding specialized chemicals to the gas stream. Another approach, known as "biofiltering," involves degrading the gases by passing them through a bed of soil, compost, or peat, where microorganisms metabolize and destroy the odor-causing chemical compounds. Table 17 lists examples of common odor-producing chemicals emitted to the atmosphere from industrial operations.

While federal agencies, such as the U.S. Environmental Protection Agency (EPA), usually do not regulate odors directly, some air pollution regulations reduce concentrations of pollutants that are also odorous, thereby indirectly preventing a community odor problem. For example, sulfur dioxide gas, which has a distinct smell and is caused by the combustion of fossil fuels at electric power plants and other industrial facilities, is subject to an EPA air quality standard that limits the amount of sulfur dioxide in the surrounding air due to health concerns.

RECOMMENDATIONS FOR CITY DWELLERS

Local health and environmental departments are interested in finding solutions to community odor problems, and organizing neighbors to file complaints with local officials can help demonstrate how widespread and serious the odor problem is. Remind public officials that because the presence of odors can sometimes indicate a more serious air pollution problem, a full investigation by the city may be called for. Another option is to

Table 17   Examples of Odor-Producing Chemicals Emitted from Industrial Operations

Odor-Producing Chemical	Industry	Characteristic Odor
Ammonia	• Fertilizer • Paper mills • Pharmaceuticals • Rubber • Semiconductors • Textiles	Sharp, pungent, suffocating odor
Benzene	• Petroleum refineries	Sweet, aromatic odor
Formaldehyde	• Coal-fired power plants • Vehicle exhaust	Strong, pungent, suffocating odor
Hydrogen sulfide	• Food processing • Landfills • Livestock feeding • Paper mills • Petroleum refineries • Wood treatment	Smells like rotten eggs
Pentachlorophenol and creosote	• Wood treatment	Pentachlorophenol—sharp, phenolic smell when hot Creosote—strong, smoky, tarlike odor
Sulfur oxides	• Coal-fired power plants • Petroleum refineries • Vehicle exhaust • Wood treatment	Sulfur-like smell, similar to a just-struck match
Toluene	• Petroleum refineries	Sweet, pungent, benzenelike odor
Xylene	• Petroleum refineries	Sweet, aromatic odor

Source: U.S. Agency for Toxic Substances and Disease Registry.

meet with the facility causing the odor to work out an amicable solution before involving the city. While waiting for a permanent solution to be implemented, urban dwellers should consider taking steps to avoid the odor by closing windows and remaining indoors or by leaving the affected area.

An effective tool for documenting odor problems is a personal odor diary. Odor diaries provide information that can help local environmental health officials identify the source of the odor and take action to reduce or eliminate the offensive smell. The information typically found in an odor diary includes the date when the odor was detected, start and end times, location, odor type and severity, effects on normal activities, weather conditions, and any comments that may be helpful in locating the source. With this information, combined with other data about air pollution emissions and air quality, local officials can identify the source of the odor, assess the severity of the problem, and formulate a solution. Try to collect several days or weeks of data so that local officials can better understand when the odors occur and what actions may be most appropriate. This information can also help the facility causing the odor to determine what remedial actions are likely to be effective.

Population Growth and Overcrowding

As the global population continues to increase in the twenty-first century, an increasing proportion of people will be living in cities, raising the specter of overcrowding in many metropolitan areas. Already, a majority of people from middle- and high-income nations are living in urban areas, and by 2050, nearly half the population of low-income countries will also be urban, as shown in Table 18. This trend toward urban growth will put an additional burden on healthcare delivery, particularly in developing nations, where many urban healthcare systems are already understaffed and lack adequate facilities. If healthcare delivery is unable to keep up with population growth, more illnesses will go untreated, and outbreaks of infectious diseases will be more difficult to control.

Many of the most rapidly growing urban areas are in China, which is no surprise, given that about one in five people on Earth live in China. Among the top 25 urban areas for population growth listed in Table 19, 10 are in China, 5 in India, 4 on the African continent, and 2 in Pakistan, and the growth rate of the fastest-growing urban area, Suzhou, China, is more than twice that of number 25, Lahore, Pakistan. Noticeably absent from the top 25 list are large cities in North and South America and Europe, most of which are growing, but at a slower rate. The population of Tokyo, by some measures the world's largest metropolitan area, is expected to grow little if any in the future as Japan's population shrinks, but this is counter to the trend of other large urban areas.

Table 18   Percent Urban Population by Income Level, 2014 and 2050

Countries' Income Level	Percent of Urban Population	
	2014	2050 (projected)
High-income countries	80	87
Middle-income countries	51	67
Low-income countries	30	48
Worldwide	54	66

Source: United Nations World Urbanization Prospects.

An unknown factor in the future growth of cities is the effect of immigration. Some countries allow immigrants to remain in the country, and even apply for citizenship under certain circumstances, and they may be granted special refugee status if escaping violence or political persecution. A number of countries also encourage seasonal migrant workers to work on farms or in the construction industry, and some migrants may remain in the country for extended periods, often relocating to urban areas to be closer to relatives. The first two decades of the twenty-first century have witnesses a refugee crisis unlike any before, where nearly 1.5 million people from war-torn areas of Syria and nearby countries risked their lives crossing the Mediterranean Sea aboard unseaworthy boats and dinghies in a desperate attempt to reach cities in Europe. Meanwhile, the United States continues to struggle with an influx of immigrants across its southern border, many seeking refugee status as they escape violence in Central America. The United Nations Refugee Agency (UNRA) reports that there are over 25 million refugees in the world—the highest number ever seen. Half of the refugees are under age 18, and two-thirds are from just five countries: Syria, Afghanistan, South Sudan, Myanmar, and Somalia.

There is growing concern among international environmental groups and world peace organizations about the potential for large-scale movements of people across political borders due to the effects of environmental degradation, especially that caused by climate change. As the earth warms due to climate change, rainfall patterns will change and deserts will expand, resulting in crop loss and famine. Also, natural disasters, such as intense storms and heat waves, will increase, infectious diseases will spread as mosquitoes and other vectors expand their territories, and coastal areas will become inundated by rising sea levels. Climate change will force masses

Table 19   Population Growth for Top 25 Urban Areas with Population Exceeding 5,000,000

Rank	City	Country	Percent Population Growth (2010–2015)
1	Suzhou	China	6.3
2	Guangzhou	China	5.2
3	Surat	India	4.8
4	Beijing	China	4.6
5	Hangzhou	China	4.6
6	Kinshasa	Congo	4.2
7	Bangalore	India	4.0
8	Ar-Riyadh (Riyadh)	Saudi Arabia	4.0
9	Luanda	Angola	4.0
10	Lagos	Nigeria	3.9
11	Chengdu	China	3.8
12	Dhaka	Bangladesh	3.6
13	Nanjing	China	3.6
14	Shanghai	China	3.4
15	Chongqing	China	3.4
16	Tianjin	China	3.4
17	Ahmadabad	India	3.4
18	Karachi	Pakistan	3.3
19	Hyderabad	India	3.3
20	Thành Pho Ho Chí Minh (Ho Chi Minh City)	Vietnam	3.3
21	Kuala Lumpur	Malaysia	3.3
22	Delhi	India	3.2
23	Johannesburg	South Africa	3.2
24	Xi'an	China	3.2
25	Lahore	Pakistan	3.1

Source: United Nations Department of Economic and Social Affairs, Population Division.

of people to leave their rural homelands just to survive, becoming urban environmental refugees. (The World Bank predicts that 140 million people could be displaced due to the effects of climate change by 2050.) According to the UNRA, "climate change will force people into increasing poverty and displacement, exacerbating the factors that lead to conflict, rendering both the humanitarian needs and responses in such situations even more complex." This dire scenario may already be taking place. Peter Maurer, head of the International Committee of the Red Cross, recently remarked, "When I think about our engagement in sub-Saharan Africa, in Somalia, in other places of the world, I see that climate change has already had a massive impact on population movement, on fertility of land."

The effects of immigration, whether due to war and violence, climate change, or simply a desire for a better life, are impossible to predict. However, it is likely that many, if not most, immigrants will move to urban areas in search of jobs and support networks consisting of others from their homeland, and experts predict that a majority of future immigrants will end up in slum areas. Increasing immigration, combined with population growth and the overall trend of people relocating to urban areas, will present an enormous burden for cities, particularly in providing healthcare services. By the middle of the century, if not sooner, dramatic changes to governance and infrastructure may be required to cope with overcrowding in many of the world's largest cities.

IMPACT ON URBAN HEALTH

When urban areas become more crowded, healthcare outcomes generally worsen, as more people compete for limited doctors and hospital beds. Additionally, there may be more cases of depression and feelings of hopelessness when people cannot readily access medical care or are forced to endure long waits in hospital emergency rooms. Quality healthcare is generally unavailable to the hundreds of millions of people living in urban slums, which is a particular concern for the future because most urban population growth in developing countries is expected to occur within slum areas. The greatest health concern in many of these areas is the spread of infectious diseases due to poor drinking water and sanitation systems.

Most big cities have improved drinking water systems, but diseases continue to be spread by these systems, particularly in overcrowded urban areas in developing countries. For example, the World Health Organization (WHO) estimates that over 50 percent of urban residents in developing countries are affected at one time or another by diseases associated with poor drinking water and inadequate sanitation, and even in developed countries, diseases are sometimes spread when drinking water becomes contaminated. Contaminated water supplies can transmit diseases like cholera, dysentery, typhoid, and polio, and worm infections from contaminated water are a particular problem in sub-Saharan Africa. Over 500,000 diarrheal deaths associated with contaminated drinking water occur globally every year.

Poor sanitation systems also plague many overcrowded developing cities, although improvements are occurring rapidly with the assistance of international aid organizations. Up to 20 percent of the global urban population continues to lack improved sanitation systems, and as many as 100 million city residents still practice open defecation, which can spread diseases and contaminate drinking-water supplies. Solid waste disposal also represents a huge problem in many cities in developing countries, where trash may accumulate in overcrowded urban areas, attracting disease-carrying rodents and insects. Despite aggressive recycling programs in some cities, steep increases in the solid waste generated by most cities around the world are predicted as populations grow while per capita waste simultaneously increases.

Water quality– and sanitation-related health problems are often worse in urban slums due to limited infrastructure, few healthcare options, and social systems that may prevent slum dwellers from improving their lives. Overcrowding exacerbates these problems by facilitating the spread of infectious diseases, such as tuberculosis, hepatitis, dengue fever, pneumonia, cholera, and malaria, and poor water quality and sanitation systems contribute to a high prevalence of diarrhea. Additionally, because of the limited healthcare afforded people living in slums, diseases like hypertension, diabetes, tuberculosis, rheumatic heart disease, and human immunodeficiency virus (HIV) infection may go untreated until late stages of the disease, leading to increased risk of stroke, myocardial infarction, kidney failure, heart valve disease, AIDS, and other complications. Table 20 shows the top 15 countries having the largest slum populations. Close to 1 billion people (one in eight people living on Earth) live in urban slums.

Ideally, as cities become more crowded, population growth would take place in a well-planned and orderly fashion so that increased traffic could be managed, public transportation options planned, and green spaces incorporated to encourage relaxation and escape from the hustle and bustle of city life. But more often than not, cities grow without good planning, resulting

Table 20   Top 15 Countries with the Largest Slum Populations

Rank	Country	Population Living in Slums	Slum Population Percent of Urban Population
1	China	191,106,700	25
2	India	98,449,000	24
3	Nigeria	42,067,100	70
4	Brazil	38,490,700	22
5	Pakistan	32,265,000	46
6	Bangladesh	29,273,000	55
7	Indonesia	29,211,800	22
8	Democratic Republic of the Congo	21,778,000	75
9	Philippines	17,055,400	38
10	Ethiopia	13,570,300	74
11	Sudan	11,939,100	92
12	Iraq	11,382,800	47
13	Mexico	10,852,000	11
14	Vietnam	8,294,600	27
15	Thailand	8,264,000	25

Source: United Nations Statistics Division.

in more stress-related ailments, including depression and anxiety, and greater exposure to air pollution. In developing nations, the use of cookstoves and open hearths (e.g., fireplaces) for cooking and heating may also increase, along with the indoor air pollution they cause, as urban areas expand and slum areas grow in size. Both outdoor and indoor air pollutants are associated with a variety of health issues, including asthma, respiratory irritation and disease, and cancer. (See the entries on "Air Quality and Urban Smog" and "Indoor Air Quality" for more information about the health effects of air pollution.)

Air pollution may become even worse in crowed urban areas as climate change increases the number and severity of heat waves (periods of several days or longer when temperatures are well above average and high enough to cause heat-related illnesses, such as heat exhaustion, heat cramps, and heatstroke). Heat waves are always worse in urban areas because of the heat island effect, which describes how the built environment warms faster and holds it heat longer than surrounding rural areas. (See the "Climate Change" and the "Green Buildings and Sustainable Development" entries to learn more about the heat island effect.) Population growth and overcrowding do not directly cause heat waves, but with more people crowding into cities at the same time that climate change is causing more warming of the earth, additional urban medical personnel and facilities will be required to address heat-related illnesses, placing a strain on city resources.

WHAT CITIES ARE DOING ABOUT POPULATION GROWTH AND OVERCROWDING

As urban populations increase, cities are responding with various policies and programs to ensure the health and safety of their citizens. To reduce the spread of infectious waterborne diseases, many cities in developing countries are focusing on water contamination from fecal matter and environmental contaminants by improving sanitation infrastructure, including better sewer systems and water treatment facilities. And, anticipating worsening air pollution in the future, cities are improving public transportation systems, increasing air pollution emission regulations for industrial and commercial operations, and requiring annual vehicle emission testing. To further reduce air pollution, some cities require industrial and commercial operations to use cleaner-burning fuels, and residents are prohibited from burning household wastes in pits in the ground or open containers, commonly 55-gallon (208-liter) drums. Reducing indoor air pollution from cookstoves and open hearths has proved to be challenging, but progress is being made with help from international aid agencies. For example, the Global Alliance for Clean Cookstoves is on track to have distributed cleaner stoves and fuels to 100 million households by 2020.

To address heat-related illnesses and reduce the mortality rate during heat waves in crowded urban areas, some cities distribute cooling fans and air conditioners to low-income residents and activate air conditioned cooling centers for public use. By paying close attention to weather forecasts, cities are improving their ability to warn the public about hot weather through public service announcements on radio and television, as well as through social media alerts. During heat-wave events, city police and fire officials sometimes check on the elderly and provide transportation to cooling centers. To further address the effects of climate change as populations grow, cities are implementing sustainability policies, such as encouraging the construction of green buildings and incorporating more trees and green spaces into the urban landscape. (For more information on sustainability in cities, see the "Green Buildings and Sustainable Development" entry.)

Another priority of cities, particularly in developing countries, is to upgrade their urban slums, where much of the future population growth within cities is expected to occur. The WHO characterizes slums as "vast islands of informal economies, social exclusion, poor housing, and underdevelopment." Cleaning up these slums while addressing economic, social, housing, and development issues is a daunting task, although some progress is being made, with the ultimate goal of transforming these areas into vibrant and healthy neighborhoods. Several positive steps that have already been put into practice in some cities include better sanitation and water-supply systems, more street paving, expanded green spaces, and improved public transportation. Also, slum residents are being mobilized to participate in the planning, management, and governance activities of their neighborhoods.

RECOMMENDATIONS FOR CITY DWELLERS

If you live in a crowded urban area or plan to visit one, these are some steps that you can take to remain healthy:

- **Water quality**—Check with city officials to learn whether the water is safe to drink. (In the United States, the State Department's Travel Advisories program maintains information on whether the tap and bottled water in the country you plan to visit are safe.) Remember that ice, frozen treats, and raw food, including fruits and vegetables, may be contaminated with waterborne pathogens, and at restaurants, be sure to check whether the food has been prepared with untreated water. Monitor yourself for symptoms of waterborne disease, such as diarrhea, vomiting, stomach cramps, and fever.

- **Air pollution**—To protect yourself from air pollution, pay attention to local air-quality alerts and remain indoors when the air quality is bad. In the United States, the Environmental Protection Agency (EPA) issues air-quality alerts through its AirNow Air Quality Index (AQI) program, and a version of this program, AirNow-International, has expanded overseas. Be aware of the early symptoms of air pollution exposure, such as an asthma episode, shortness of breath, wheezing, chest pain, headache, nausea, or fatigue.

- **Heat-related illnesses**—On unusually hot days, drink plenty of water and remain indoors in air conditioned spaces as much as possible. Close the blinds and curtains during the hottest parts of the day, and open windows when temperatures cool off in the evening. While outside, wear lightweight, light-colored clothing and stay in shady areas. If there is no air conditioning where you are, visit a cooling center or a public facility like a movie theater or shopping mall. Watch for symptoms of dehydration and heat stress, including muscle cramps, headaches, dizziness, and fatigue.

- **Climate change**—To help fight climate change, take public transportation whenever possible or drive an electric or hybrid automobile, and avoid wasting energy (e.g., turn lights off when not in use, wash clothes in cold water and hang them up to dry, and cut back some on your home's heating or air conditioning.) Support environmental activist groups promoting renewable energy, green buildings, and public transportation, and consider voting for candidates who support programs to reduce climate change.

By taking these precautions, you can protect your health while still enjoying the many benefits of city life.

CITY SPOTLIGHT: KARACHI—GLIMMERS OF HOPE FOR THE WORLD'S LARGEST SLUM

It is hard to be optimistic about the future of the world's growing slum areas, including the part of Karachi known as Orangi Town. But self-help programs and the empowerment of slum dwellers to solve their own problems may lead the way toward a brighter future.

Over 900 million people live in urban slums worldwide, and that number is expected to grow to as many as one in four people on Earth by 2030. These slum dwellers often subsist under the worst possible conditions—large families living in one- or two-room shacks with no plumbing or electricity, surrounded by neighborhood landfills or waste dumps and with sewage flowing through the streets. Health professionals speak of a cycle of poverty in slum areas, where workers are marginalized due to ethnic barriers and lack of a permanent home address, poor nutrition leaves residents vulnerable to infectious diseases, and children frequently miss school due to illness, if they are lucky enough to go to school at all. Up to 90 percent of urbanization this century will occur within slums, as migrants to cities from poor rural areas lack the resources to live anywhere else.

The world's largest slum is an area called Orangi Town, which is in Karachi, Pakistan. No one knows exactly how many people live in Orangi Town, but current estimates place the population at around 2.4 million—about the same size as Houston, Texas, the fourth-largest U.S. city. However, the population density of Orangi Town is many times that of Houston, ranking it among the most densely populated areas in the world. Today, Orangi Town is home to a booming cottage industry, making slippers, saris, and other items sold in Karachi and sometimes exported.

Orangi Town is different from many other slum areas, in that housing is not the primary concern. Most families' homes are small structures housing 8–10 people, consisting of no more than two or three tiny rooms built from concrete blocks manufactured locally. A greater problem in Orangi Town has been the lack of basic services, particularly potable water, which is in very short supply. The water situation is so bad that women are forced to walk long distances in the hope of finding a little water to fill their water jugs, and some farmers on the edge of town can only access water mixed with sewage. The area also suffers from rampant street crime and ethnic clashes, a critical shortage of schools and hospitals, child labor issues, and corruption that illegally channels precious water to factories.

Basic sanitation, including a sewer system, was absent from Orangi Town for many years, and residents often complained of raw sewage being everywhere. In the 1980s, when it became apparent that the Karachi city government would not help remedy this problem, local residents took it upon themselves to design, finance, and build an extensive sewer system that today provides service to most streets. This success story was made possible by the Orangi Pilot Project, a self-help scheme started by the legendary Dr. Akhtar Hamid Khan that empowered residents to solve their own problems. (Dr. Khan pioneered many innovative methods for alleviating poverty that have had a worldwide influence.) Following the pilot project, residents made great strides in putting in water pipes, building schools and health clinics, and improving roads. Nevertheless, the area remains desperately poor, with too few doctors and a thriving quack-doctor industry that does more harm than good.

The 2018 heat wave was particularly hard on Orangi Town, when temperatures reached 111°F (44°C). With no air conditioning and fans operating only during the few hours each day when the electricity was on, people stayed indoors as much as possible, relying on wet washcloths for some relief from the heat. Because the heat wave occurred during the Muslim holy month of Ramadan, when many Muslims abstain from food and water from sunrise to sunset, the struggle against the heat was especially difficult. The number of heat-related deaths is unknown, but a similar heat wave in 2015 is believed to have killed over 1,000 people, and tens of thousands reportedly suffered from heat stress and related conditions.

According to the WHO, living in an urban setting can be a social determinant for poor health, particularly in slum areas like Orangi Town. For the one-third of the world's urban population living in slums, disease is rampant, especially infectious diseases such as tuberculosis, hepatitis, dengue fever, pneumonia, cholera, and malaria. There is also a high prevalence of diarrhea, and with little or no air conditioning and few shade trees, slum areas suffer disproportionately from heat waves. The WHO reports that over 90 percent of the world's urban population, including most of the people residing in urban slums, is exposed to air pollution worse than WHO health guideline limits, and indoor air pollution from the use of poorly ventilated cookstoves in homes causes about 3.8 million premature deaths annually.

Urbanization has helped millions of people escape poverty and find a better life. But too often, cities have been unable or unwilling to provide socioeconomic and cultural opportunities for all of their citizens, as well as the physical infrastructure needed for the poorest residents to live with dignity and hope. Instead, the disparities between urban rich and poor appear to be growing, with 75 percent of the world's cities having higher levels of income inequality than two decades ago, according to the United Nations. The self-help model pioneered in Orangi Town is a promising approach to addressing urban poverty and an exciting new way of thinking, but as the number of poor urban dwellers this century continues to grow, a stronger commitment from cities and nations will be needed to alleviate the suffering and provide equal opportunities for all.

EXPERT COMMENTARY: IMMIGRANT HEALTH AND SAFETY

One common misconception, often invoked in immigration debates, is that immigration increases the risk of communicable diseases in destination countries.

Georgiana Bostean, Assistant Professor

Chapman University

Dr. Bostean is an assistant professor of Environment, Health, and Policy at Chapman University. She is an expert in population health disparities, specializing in cancer-related health behaviors, including tobacco use. Her research has been supported by grants from the National Science Foundation (NSF) and published in several scientific journals, including the American Journal of Public Health *and* Social Science and Medicine.

What do you see as the greatest issues regarding immigrant health and safety in urban areas, what are the major obstacles to addressing these issues, and what is your hope for the future?

An estimated 258 million people live in a country other than their country of birth—an increase of 49 percent since 2000, according to the *International Migration Report.* The health and safety issues facing immigrants in urban areas are complex and determined by a plethora of factors, including conditions in the migrant's country of origin, the migration circumstances (whether voluntary or forced, and experiences during migration), and the reception and integration in the destination country and society.

The bulk of global migrants go to high-income countries, where immigration is an increasingly politicized issue. One common misconception, often invoked in immigration debates, is that immigration increases the risk of communicable diseases in destination countries. However, evidence shows that migrants do not pose an increased threat for the spread of infectious diseases. On the contrary, immigration has benefited population health in some countries by slowing population aging and decline. In many high-income countries (e.g., in Europe, North America, and Australia), immigrants have lower mortality rates and better health than the native-born populations, despite coming from socioeconomically disadvantaged countries—a phenomenon called the "healthy immigrant effect" or "immigrant health paradox."

However, immigrants' health tends to deteriorate the longer they live in their host countries. Immigrants face many of the same health challenges as the native-born, but their health problems may be exacerbated. For instance, for migrants facing a chronic health condition, migration can cause an interruption in care, which leads to health deterioration. Factors such as a lack of access to healthcare, poor working and living conditions, social exclusion due to xenophobia or discrimination (or both) in the host community, separation from family, and other social determinants may contribute to immigrants' negative health trajectories in their host countries.

As evidence mounts about how social determinants affect health, it is increasingly clear that health is shaped by all policies, not just health policy. Therefore, migrant-inclusive policies are needed to protect immigrant health. Of utmost importance is immigration policy, as legal status affects all aspects of migrants' experiences and outcomes, from the conditions under which they migrate (being more likely to undertake perilous clandestine migration journeys in the absence of legal routes of entry) to their access to health services. Immigration will continue to shape population health globally into the twenty-first century, making it imperative to adopt evidence-based policies and approaches to immigrant integration to protect the health of both immigrants and their host-country populations.

Radiation Sources

Radiation—energy in the form of electromagnetic waves or subatomic particles—is all around us in the urban environment. Radio waves, microwaves, and visible light are examples of radiation, as are X-rays and cosmic particles from outer space. Most of the radiation that we are exposed to comes from background sources (e.g., from outer space and from naturally occurring radioactive minerals found in the soil and water). Ultraviolet (UV) radiation from the sun is another type of radiation that we are exposed to every time we step outside. We can also be exposed to radiation from certain medical diagnostic equipment, radiation therapy, research and manufacturing technologies, and accidents at nuclear power plants. Most radiation is harmless, but some types can threaten our health, potentially causing radiation sickness, cancer, and other illnesses.

When we consider the various health risks associated with city living, we usually do not think about radiation. After all, we cannot see, hear, or smell radiation, and we seldom learn of someone sickened from it. Nevertheless, there are several types of radiation in urban areas that we need to pay attention to if we want to stay healthy and avoid potentially dangerous exposure. The greatest concern is about radon gas, which can concentrate in homes and other buildings. Additionally, some scientists caution about overexposure to certain types of electromagnetic radiation, and UV radiation from the sun can also be a concern, even in the city. People living near a nuclear power plant should be prepared to follow evacuation orders in the unlikely event of an accidental release of radioactive gas.

There are two types of radiation: ionizing and nonionizing. Ionizing radiation is strong enough to dislodge electrons from their atomic orbits, causing the atom to become charged (i.e., ionized). Ionizing radiation can damage tissues, alter the deoxyribonucleic acid (DNA) in genes, and sometimes cause cancer. (Because cancers are slow to develop, the effects of chronic exposure to ionizing radiation may not be apparent for 20 years or longer.) Also, exposure to high levels of ionizing radiation over a short period can cause radiation sickness, and even death, if there is significant damage to bone marrow, the gastrointestinal tract, or the central nervous system.

In contrast to ionizing radiation, nonionizing radiation is not powerful enough to dislodge electrons. Nonionizing radiation excites atoms (i.e., causes them to move around and vibrate), resulting in an increase in temperature, such as in the way a microwave oven thaws a frozen dinner and warms leftovers. The background levels of nonionizing radiation, which are always around us, are generally harmless. However, there is some controversy about whether long-term exposure to some nonionizing radiation sources, such as high-power electric transmission lines and cell phones, represents a health risk. It is more certain, however, that occupational exposure to high levels of nonionizing radiation (e.g., laser light and high-intensity radio waves and microwaves) can lead to harmful health effects. Table 21 presents examples of ionizing and nonionizing radiation.

All radiation travels through empty space at the same speed, about 186,000 miles per second (3.0×10^8 meters per second), but radiation types differ according to their wavelength (which is inversely proportional to

Table 21   Examples of Ionizing and Nonionizing Radiation

Ionizing	Nonionizing
Alpha particles	Extremely low-frequency radiation
Beta particles	Radio waves
Gamma rays	Microwaves
X-rays	Laser beams
Neutrons	Infrared radiation
	Visible light spectrum
	UV radiation[a]

[a]UV radiation is usually classified as nonionizing, although it can sometimes cause harmful health effects similar to ionizing radiation (e.g., damaging DNA molecules and increasing the risk of cancer).

frequency) and energy. Ionizing radiation has a shorter wavelength than nonionizing radiation, which means that there is a higher frequency of waves passing a point in space over a given time frame. In contrast, non-ionizing radiation has a longer wavelength and lower frequency. Higher-frequency waves can impart more energy, which explains why exposure to ionizing radiation represents a greater health risk.

The health risk from radiation exposure is often difficult to predict. This is because the health effects depend on a number of factors, such as the type of radiation, level and duration of exposure, target organs receiving the most exposure, overall health and age of the exposed individual, cumulative exposure over time, and time delay before certain effects become evident. The prediction of ill health from radiation exposure is a complex task, but there is extensive research in this area, and medical experts are highly trained to determine the best treatments for specific exposure scenarios.

IMPACT ON URBAN HEALTH

As previously stated, the most common radiation concern in cities is radon, which is a radioactive gas that forms naturally from the decay of radioactive elements found in soil and rock. When buildings are constructed using radon-emitting material (e.g., rock, brick, gypsum, or concrete) or located above soil containing radioactive elements, radon gases can enter the structure and concentrate in living spaces, potentially building up to levels high enough to harm us. Radon exposure is primarily associated with lung cancer, and it is the second-leading cause of lung cancer in the United States. According to the World Health Organization (WHO), radon exposure at home or on the job is one of the main risks from ionizing radiation, resulting in tens of thousands of lung cancer deaths annually throughout the world. (Only tobacco smoking results in more lung cancer deaths.) Radon can accumulate in all types of buildings, but the greatest exposure often occurs at home because we spend so much of our time there—more so than at work or school.

If you live in the city, you are surrounded by electromagnetic fields (EMFs)—electrical and magnetic energy associated with electrical devices, residential wiring, power lines and cables, home appliances, and any other device that carries electrical current. Most experts believe the low levels of EMFs that we are commonly exposed to are of little or no concern. Much of the early research on health effects focused on extremely low-frequency EMF from electric power sources, including power lines, electrical substations, and certain home appliances. Some of these studies revealed a possible link between EMF and childhood leukemia, but the associations were weak. More recent studies examining devices such as cell phones, wireless routers, and global positioning system (GPS) devices similarly found weak (if any) association. Several studies have found no evidence of association between EMF and adult cancers, including leukemia and brain and breast cancers.

Based on these studies, the WHO has concluded that, given the weakness of the evidence for childhood leukemia, the benefits of EMF exposure reduction on health are unclear. Similarly, the U.S. Environmental Protection Agency (EPA) has determined that scientific studies have not clearly shown whether exposure to EMF increases cancer risk. On the other hand, the International Agency for Research on Cancer has placed radio-frequency electromagnetic fields into Group 2B, "Possibly Carcinogenic to Humans," "based on an increased risk for glioma, a malignant type of brain cancer, associated with wireless phone use." Research on EMF is ongoing, and the U.S. National Institute of Environmental Health Sciences recommends continued education on practical ways to reduce EMF exposure.

UV radiation from the sun is a form of radiation that causes sunburn. We tend to worry most about sunburn while on vacation at the beach, and sometimes we forget that sunburn can just as easily occur in the city while walking to work, enjoying lunch in the park, or working in a garden. The sunburn that we get in the city can actually be worse than on vacation because we may not take the same precautions to protect ourselves, such as wearing sunscreen lotion and a hat.

UV exposure varies widely among the world's cities, depending on a number of factors. For example, cities having a higher elevation and lower latitude (i.e., closer to the equator) tend to have more days with higher UV Index values. (The UV Index scale, presented in Table 22, is used to forecast the risk of excessive exposure to UV radiation from the sun, where higher index values represent greater risk.) Cities in the Southern Hemisphere tend to have higher UV indices due to the stratospheric ozone hole (i.e., the seasonal depletion of the ozone layer over the South Pole due to air pollution), which allows more UV radiation to reach the earth's surface. Other factors include climate and the presence of sand, snow, or water, which can reflect UV radiation and intensify exposure. Because of these

Table 22   UV Index Scale

UV Index	Category	Precautions
0–2	Low (Green)	A UV Index reading of 0–2 means low danger from the sun's UV rays for the average person. Wear sunglasses on bright days. If you burn easily, cover up and use broad-spectrum, SPF 30+ sunscreen. Watch out for bright surfaces, like sand, water, and snow, which reflect UV and increase exposure.
3–5	Moderate (Yellow)	A UV Index reading of 3–5 means moderate risk of harm from unprotected sun exposure. Stay in the shade near midday, when the sun is strongest. If outdoors, wear protective clothing, a wide-brimmed hat, and UV-blocking sunglasses. Generously apply broad-spectrum, SPF 30+ sunscreen every 2 hours, even on cloudy days, and after swimming or sweating. Watch out for bright surfaces, like sand, water, and snow, which reflect UV and increase exposure.
6–7	High (Orange)	A UV Index reading of 6–7 means high risk of harm from unprotected sun exposure. Protection against skin and eye damage is needed. Reduce time in the sun between 10 a.m. and 4 p.m. If outdoors, seek shade and wear protective clothing, a wide-brimmed hat, and UV-blocking sunglasses. Generously apply broad-spectrum, SPF 30+ sunscreen every 2 hours, even on cloudy days, and after swimming or sweating. Watch out for bright surfaces, like sand, water, and snow, which reflect UV and increase exposure.
8–10	Very High (Red)	A UV Index reading of 8–10 means very high risk of harm from unprotected sun exposure. Take extra precautions because unprotected skin and eyes will be damaged and can burn quickly.

Table 22   (continued)

UV Index	Category	Precautions
		Minimize sun exposure between 10 a.m. and 4 p.m. If outdoors, seek shade and wear protective clothing, a wide-brimmed hat, and UV-blocking sunglasses. Generously apply broad-spectrum, SPF 30+ sunscreen every 2 hours, even on cloudy days, and after swimming or sweating. Watch out for bright surfaces, like sand, water, and snow, which reflect UV and increase exposure.
11 or more	Extreme (Purple)	A UV Index reading of 11 or more means extreme risk of harm from unprotected sun exposure. Take all precautions because unprotected skin and eyes can burn in minutes. Try to avoid sun exposure between 10 a.m. and 4 p.m. If outdoors, seek shade and wear protective clothing, a wide-brimmed hat, and UV-blocking sunglasses. Generously apply broad-spectrum, SPF 30+ sunscreen every 2 hours, even on cloudy days, and after swimming or sweating. Watch out for bright surfaces, like sand, water, and snow, which reflect UV and increase exposure.

Source: EPA.

factors, some cities typically have higher UV index values than others. The WHO has calculated representative maximal UV index values (which vary by month) for a number of cities, including those listed in Table 23.

Among the health consequences of overexposure to UV radiation, skin cancer is perhaps the most serious. However, excessive UV radiation exposure can also cause "actinic keratoses," which are growths of skin on overexposed areas of the body (especially the face, hands, neck, and forearms) that are risk factors for later development of cancer. Additionally, premature aging of the skin can occur, making the skin look old and wrinkled. Overexposure to UV radiation can also cause reddening of the skin (erythema), reduced vitamin D synthesis, cataracts, and suppression of the

Table 23   Maximal UV Index Values

City	January	July
Bangkok	8	12
Berlin	1	7
Buenos Aires	9	2
Cape Town	9	3
Los Angeles	3	10
Melbourne	8	2
Nairobi	12	11
New York	2	9
Panama City	9	12
Paris	1	7
Rio de Janeiro	12	5
Singapore	11	11
St. Petersburg	0	5
Tokyo	2	10
Vancouver	1	7

immune system. Several types of medications may make the skin more photosensitive to UV radiation, and some medical conditions can also increase sun sensitivity.

Millions of people throughout the world live in cities close enough to a nuclear power plant to be exposed to radiation from an accident, particularly if there is an explosion that spreads radioactive gas and dust over a wide area. While this is highly unlikely, incidents at the Chernobyl nuclear plant in Ukraine (1986) and Fukushima Daiichi plant in Japan (2011) demonstrate that accidents can and do happen, requiring evacuations of nearby cities. Following evacuation orders is essential because exposure to high levels of radiation following a nuclear power plant accident can cause serious, life-threatening health issues, including radiation sickness.

The initial symptoms of radiation sickness include nausea and vomiting, sometimes accompanied by headache, diarrhea, and fever, and usually the higher the exposure level, the sooner these symptoms appear. Following the initial symptoms, there may be a brief period when no new symptoms appear, followed by the onset of new symptoms that may be more serious, such as loss of appetite, fatigue, dizziness, and even seizures and coma. Symptoms may occur within minutes or days after exposure, and they may come and go. With high doses, damage to the skin may be apparent, including swelling, itching, redness, and even blisters and ulcers. Skin damage may appear within a few hours of exposure or be delayed several days. When death occurs, the cause is typically due to the destruction of bone marrow, which results in infections and internal bleeding.

In addition to radiation sickness, exposure to high levels of radiation from a nuclear plant or industrial accident can cause other serious health conditions. These include cataracts, sterility, and fetal effects. Many survivors of the World War II atomic bomb attacks on Hiroshima and Nagasaki, Japan, experienced often fatal symptoms of radiation sickness, along with disfiguring keloid scars, sterility, birth defects, psychosomatic disorders, cataracts, leukemia, and cancers of the thyroid gland, breast, lung, and salivary glands.

Did you know that the food we buy at our local grocery store is sometimes irradiated? By briefly exposing food to radiation, such as gamma rays, X-rays, or electron beams, spoilage can be delayed, shelf life extended, disease-causing microbes reduced, and sprouting inhibited. Additionally, disinfestation can be achieved without the need for chemical insecticides. (Irradiation does not eliminate dangerous toxins already in food and does not stop fruits and vegetables from aging.) Irradiated food is safe because it does not come into contact with radiation sources, and the radiation itself cannot make food radioactive. (Similarly, the X-rays we receive at our dentist's office do not give us radioactive teeth.) Furthermore, there is relatively little difference in quality between irradiated and nonirradiated foods, although the flavor of some irradiated foods may be slightly altered. A variety of foods can be irradiated, including herbs and spices, fresh fruits and vegetables, wheat and flour, pork and poultry, red meats, and some seafood.

WHAT CITIES ARE DOING ABOUT RADIATION SOURCES

Many large cities have radiological health departments that regulate radioactive materials used in the city for academic, research, and medical purposes, including the use of medical diagnostic equipment. Cities may license such uses and perform inspections to ensure that facilities protect the health and safety of patients, employees, and the general public. Additionally, city water departments ensure that there are safe levels of radionuclides in drinking water, and some cities have radon mitigation programs to help residents and businesses assess and mitigate radon problems. These mitigation programs may include monitoring and remediation guidelines, technical support, and financial loans. Cities and states also establish emergency response plans in case there is an unexpected release of radioactive gas during a nuclear power plant accident.

Larger cities are also equipped to handle emergency situations involving radiation, such as from an accidental spill of radioactive materials while in transport or from a terrorist incident. These situations may be addressed by local fire departments or specialized hazardous materials teams, where the response may include radiological surveys of areas suspected of having radioactive contamination and the remediation of contaminated sites.

RECOMMENDATIONS FOR CITY DWELLERS

It is a good idea for people to check their homes for radon, and test kits are inexpensive and readily available. If a radon problem is discovered, it is best to hire an expert who specializes in radon remediation. A common technique for reducing radon concentrations is to install a soil suction radon reduction system, which essentially consists of vent pipes and fans that pull radon from beneath the building and vent it to the outside air. And by sealing foundation cracks and other openings in the foundation and basement, this system will work even better. Other techniques are also available, and a radon expert can provide advice about the best system for each specific situation.

Because new homes are often well sealed to be energy efficient, radon concentrations can build up. Many such homes include radon mitigation systems during construction as a precaution, particularly if located in regions known to have radon problems. To protect new homes from radon, the EPA recommends the following low-cost steps during construction: (1) install a layer of clean gravel or aggregate below the slab or flooring system; (2) lay a polyethylene sheet on top of the gravel or aggregate layer; (3) install a venting pipe from the gravel level through the building to the roof; and (4) seal and caulk the foundation carefully.

People concerned about EMF can purchase an EMF meter to measure individual exposure, or they can ask the local power company to make an on-site reading. The strength of EMF drops off quickly as a person moves away from the source, and thus, distancing oneself from the source is the best approach to reducing exposure. Because cell phones are in such widespread use, particularly by young adults whose bodies are still developing, some experts recommend reducing exposure to cell-phone EMF by (1) using the built-in speaker or a hands-free device, which will keep the phone farther from the head; (2) making fewer calls and having shorter conversations; (3) using text messaging (texting) instead of talking; (4) making calls in good reception areas, which allow the phone to transmit at reduced power; and (5) buying a phone with a lower specific absorption rate (SAR). Additional expert information on cell phones and your health is available at the websites of the Centers for Disease Control and Prevention (CDC; https://www.cdc.gov/nceh/radiation/cell_phones._faq.html) and WHO (https://www.who.int/en/news-room/fact-sheets/detail/electromagnetic-fields-and-public-health-mobile-phones).

If you are concerned about overexposure to UV radiation while outdoors, the following actions will help you avoid getting too much harmful sunlight:

- Limiting time spent in the midday sun, especially during the hours from 10:00 a.m. to 4:00 p.m.
- Applying a broad-spectrum, SPF 30+ sunscreen before going outside, and reapplying it frequently.
- Avoiding sunburn, which can significantly increase the risk of developing skin cancer. (You can get a sunburn even on a cloudy day!)
- Staying in the shade as much as possible while outside.
- Being careful near water, snow, and sand, which can reflect sunlight and increase the risk of sunburn.
- Wearing wide-brimmed hats, tightly woven, loose-fitting clothing, and sunglasses that provide 100 percent UV protection against both UVA and UVB radiation.
- Checking the UV Index before planning outdoor activities to be sure that you are adequately protected.

Additionally, read the warning labels on any medications to determine if they can make the skin more photosensitive to UV radiation. And stay away from sunbeds, sunlamps, and tanning booths, which can increase the risks of sunburn, accelerated skin aging, eye inflammation, immune system suppression, and melanoma and nonmelanoma skin cancer. (The WHO reports that when the first use of a sunbed occurs before age 35, the risk of developing melanoma increases by 59 percent.) Finally, people should examine their skin at least monthly, looking for abnormalities, such as moles that have changed size, color, or shape and sores that have not healed.

Nuclear power plants are highly regulated and seldom experience accidents. However, if you live near a nuclear power plant, are you prepared for the worst-case scenario—

the release of dangerous radiation that spreads in your direction? There are steps that individuals and families should take to be prepared. For example, have an emergency supply kit that contains all the items needed in case of evacuation, including medical prescriptions and supplies and important documents. Additionally, develop a family emergency plan that contains information on what to do, how to contact family members, and where to meet during an emergency. Knowing the local evacuation routes is also a good idea, and be sure to bring your pets. Check with the local emergency response office for specific recommendations for the city you live in.

Social Support Networks

Life is full of challenges, and sometimes unexpected events like the loss of a job or death of a loved one can leave you feeling alone and helpless, not knowing where to turn for moral support and assistance. At other times, you may need help arranging care for an older parent or planning an important event like a wedding. A "social support network" consists of friends, family, coworkers, and others in your community who you can turn to in times of need, and likewise, they may seek your support as challenges arise in their own lives. Having a social support network can have wide-ranging benefits for your health and well-being.

Social support networks are particularly effective in coping with the stress of urban life, and many city residents have found that having a network in place before issues occur is almost like having an insurance policy to protect against the unexpected. A social support network is usually not a formal group with regular meetings; instead, it tends to be a loose collection of people that you know you can count on. Making time to cultivate relationships and build a strong support network may be one of the smartest steps that you can take to survive and thrive in the city.

A social support network is not the same as a "support group," which has a specific objective and often takes the form of a structured meeting run by a mental health professional or social worker. An example of a support group is a weekly meeting of people having alcohol problems, led by a counselor trained in alcohol abuse intervention. In contrast, a social support network is built up over time as bonds with friends and family are strengthened through interactions at home, work, school, or religious services.

In addition to providing someone to talk with when problems arise, simply having a social support network in place has been shown to have important psychological benefits. Knowing there are others in your network who care about you—whom you can turn to in times of need—can provide a sense of belonging and self-worth and a feeling of security. And when people reach out to *you* in their times of need, you may feel like a more valued member of society. By helping people cope with the challenges of daily life in a busy city environment, including the social isolation experienced by many urban residents, social support networks support good mental health and help prevent the onset of stress-related illness.

While most social support networks are informal, support networks sometimes take on a more organized structure, particularly if the network provides specialized services to specific ethnic or cultural groups. One example is the Vietnamese Community Health Initiative in New York City. A top priority for this support network is providing improved healthcare for the rapidly growing Vietnamese population of the city, where almost one-third of Vietnamese have no health insurance and live below the poverty level, half of young Vietnamese adults do not know enough about HIV/AIDS to protect themselves, and 90 percent of elderly Vietnamese speak little or no English.

Another example of a more structured social support network is a collection of support groups known as the Village Movement. Villages are nonprofit, grassroots, membership-based organizations that serve as social support networks for older adults living in a community or town. Villages provide the services and social interactions necessary for older adults to age independently while living at home through such aids as transportation to medical appointments, assistance with grocery shopping, help operating computers and other electronics, and opportunities to attend social events with like-minded individuals. By supporting the needs of older adults living in the neighborhood, Villages have a significant impact on the social determinants of health for a city's older adults. There are over 200 Villages across the United States and in several other countries, and while each Village is an independent organization, many of them belong to the Village-to-Village Network, an umbrella organization providing guidance, resources, and support.

IMPACT ON URBAN HEALTH

Research involving the benefits of social support networks to health has generally found that high levels of social support are positively correlated with good physical and mental health and longevity in populations as diverse as college students, unemployed workers, and new mothers. Positive social interactions can improve motivation when being around people with the same goals (e.g., losing weight), and the support and encouragement received from family and friends in your network can encourage healthy choices and behaviors, such as having a good diet, exercising regularly, and avoiding tobacco and drugs. Furthermore, support networks help reduce stress-related illnesses by being around people who your health and well-being.

On the other hand, poor social support is associated with loneliness, which is known to increase the risk of depression, suicide, alcohol use, and cardiovascular disease. Also, research suggests that poor social support is correlated with reduced life expectancy, and this correlation may be as strong as the effects of obesity, tobacco smoking, hypertension, and lack of physical activity on longevity.

Ongoing research on social support networks has uncovered some interesting results, including the following:

- Social isolation is a major risk factor for illness, while having a strong social support network can have the opposite effect—reducing illness and improving quality of life.
- Both men and women lacking strong social support networks may be up to three times more likely to die from a variety of ailments, including ischemic heart disease, cerebral vascular disease, and cancer, compared with individuals having more social contact.
- Poor social support is associated with depression and other mood disorders, including depression occurring among patients suffering from other diseases such as cancer. However, having a strong social support network may decrease functional impairment and increase recovery in patients with depression.
- Within a social support network, the *quality* of social interactions appears to be more important for one's health and well-being than the *quantity* of interactions. Perhaps this is obvious, but having a few very close friends that you can always count on and confide in is more important than having a larger network of people where the bonds of friendship and trust are not as strong.
- For military personnel having experienced combat trauma, strong social support may reduce the risk of developing posttraumatic stress disorder (PTSD).

A considerable amount of research has been conducted on American soldiers returning from the unpopular Vietnam War, which ended in 1975. Upon arriving home, these servicemen and servicewomen often had little or no support network and felt alone and rejected, particularly by younger people (often their peers) who protested the war and burned their military draft registration cards in protest. Among soldiers who experienced PTSD, homecoming stress was found to be a strong predictor of the frequency and intensity of their symptoms. These soldiers almost certainly would have benefited from strong social support networks, with friends and loved ones available to help them adjust to their new life at home.

When on the giving end of a relationship, as opposed to the receiving end, there can also be substantial benefits. For example, one study found that providing support to others lowered blood pressure, and in another study, older adults who felt socially useful to others experienced lower disability and mortality. In a survey, people who provided support to someone else in a social support network reported that they were more likely to receive support in return when needed.

While social networks provide unquestioned benefits to a community, there can be circumstances where they are not helpful, even possibly becoming a hindrance. For example, research shows that in some urban-area ethnic communities, older parents are reluctant to ask their grown-up children, who are busy working and raising their own families, for help getting to medical appointments or the drugstore. At the same time, they may not call on others in their social network for assistance, apparently over concern about what others will think if they cannot rely on their children. The result is that older parents in some ethnic communities do not seek medical attention as often as they should. Other research shows that inadequate or misguided help from social network members (e.g., urging the use of home or ethnic remedies) can deter optimal health service use, and as a consequence, some minority groups have a tendency to present themselves to health professionals during the later stages of illness. And in some cases, associating with a network of individuals making poor choices, like drug use, may encourage others in the network to do the same.

Much more research is needed to fully understand all of the benefits and drawbacks of belonging to a social support network, but one fact is clear: For most people, positive and supportive social support networks are good for both physical and mental health and may even increase longevity for both the giver and the receiver of support.

WHAT CITIES ARE DOING ABOUT SOCIAL SUPPORT NETWORKS

Cities provide a wide range of services that bring networks of people together to address common concerns. For example, a health agency may sponsor a focus group for recovering alcoholics, or a social services department may provide nutrition counseling and support for families living in poverty. Recognizing the power of social support networks, cities also promote and encourage support networks through programs designed to bring people together to solve local problems. For example, city officials might organize a citizens' commission to address the drug abuse prevalent in one part of town, or a town council member might form a task force to look into lead poisoning among children living in poverty. Similarly, a citywide workgroup might engage city residents in an examination of the problems of poor nutrition and high infant mortality among certain ethnic or immigrant populations. By reaching out to their own social support networks, the citizens involved with such commissions, task forces, and workgroups can distribute educational materials and gather important analytical data.

The networks of relationships among people who live and work in a city, sometimes called "social capital," are a vital part of a healthy community and necessary for cities to function effectively. Social networks are particularly important in promoting better health, lowering crime rates, improving access to city services, and building trust in elected officials. Unfortunately, there is evidence that social capital is diminishing in many cities, as fewer people participate in civic organizations and other social groups and as trust in the political process is declining. The modern-day demands of working and raising a family in the city may leave people exhausted at the end of the day, with little time or incentive for social network–expanding activities.

Most city officials agree that if their cities are to remain strong and vibrant, more must be done to strengthen social networks. To address this concern, some cities have turned to innovative urban designs to encourage human interactions. For example, pedestrian malls can be designed specifically for local businesses having ties with the surrounding community, and unused or abandoned buildings can be converted into community centers that provide meeting rooms for community discussions. Parks, sidewalks, city squares, and urban furniture can also stimulate human interactions and increase the vitality of a city. Research shows that when long, uninteresting building facades extending across city blocks are replaced with storefronts, coffee shops, and restaurants, and when narrow sidewalks are replaced with wide, walkable areas incorporating trees and benches, people slow down their pace and stop to talk.

Many cities also build networks of concerned citizens through social media. One popular U.S. social media platform, Nextdoor, allows people to share information about events or concerns in their neighborhoods, and cities often tap into this system to distribute information from their health, planning, or public safety departments. Cities also encourage and support nonprofit agencies like Meals on Wheels, a public-private partnership that helps address loneliness and isolation among older people by scheduling frequent visits by volunteers providing meals. (For many older people, Meals on Wheels provides their only daily human contact.) Some cities help put residents in touch with charitable and social organizations through clearinghouses and hotlines.

Cohousing developments within cities, where permitted by zoning codes, can be particularly effective in promoting social interaction and support. These are intentional communities usually consisting of private homes, condominiums, or apartments clustered around a shared space, which may include gardens, walkways, and a common house for periodic communal meals, meetings, and events. Cohousing residents collectively plan social activities, such as parties, games, and movies, and while there are many types of cohousing communities, they all share the common goal of promoting social interaction and support for their members.

RECOMMENDATIONS FOR CITY DWELLERS

Creating a social support network needs to be a priority in one's life, and it is a mistake to wait for someone else to make the first move. There is no reason to be shy about asking a friend to meet at the local coffee shop or inviting the neighbors over for dinner. If you have difficulty making new friends, consider getting to know people through volunteer work or religious organizations, or possibly there is someone at school or work who is just as anxious as you to develop a friendship. Sometimes reaching out to family members can be difficult, particularly if there have been communication issues in the past. But making an effort to strengthen family ties can be valuable because family members know you best and are more likely to respond in times of need. Table 24 provides some suggestions from the American Psychological Association for growing a social support network.

Remember that it takes two to build a successful friendship, and you need to do your part to nourish the relationship. Some good habits are returning phone calls and responding to emails quickly, being a good listener, complimenting friends on their successes, and showing sympathy with their troubles. On the other hand, be careful not to annoy people by being too pushy or assertive, and stay away from people who have negative attitudes or are involved with unhealthy behaviors like drug abuse. Also, avoid spending too much time online at social media sites because

Table 24   Tips for Growing a Social Support Network

Tip	Description
Cast a wide net.	When it comes to your social supports, one size doesn't fit all. You may not have one single person you can confide in about everything—and that's OK. Maybe you have a colleague you can talk to about problems at work, and a neighbor who listens to you when you have difficulties with your kids. Look to different relationships to provide different kinds of support. But remember to look to people you can trust and count on in order to avoid disappointing, negative interactions that can make you feel worse.
Be proactive.	Often, people expect others to reach out to them and then feel rejected when people don't go out of their way to do so. To get the most out of your social relationships, you have to make an effort. Make time for friends and family. Reach out to lend a hand or just say hello. If you're there for others, they'll be more likely to be there for you. And in fact, when it comes to longevity, research suggests that giving social support to friends and family may be even more important than receiving it.
Take advantage of technology.	It's nice to sit down with a friend face to face, but it isn't always possible. Luckily, technology makes it easier than ever before to stay connected with loved ones far away. Write an email, send a text message, or make a date for a video chat. Don't rely too heavily on digital connections, however. Some research suggests that face-to-face interactions are the most beneficial.
Follow your interests.	Do you like to hike, sing, make jewelry, play tennis, or get involved in local politics? You're more likely to connect with people who like the things you like. Join a club, sign up for a class, or take on a volunteer position that will allow you to meet others who share your interests. Don't be discouraged if you don't make friends overnight. Try to enjoy the experience as you get to know others over time.

(continued)

Table 24   (continued)

Tip	Description
Seek out peer support.	If you're dealing with a specific stressful situation—such as caring for a family member or dealing with a chronic illness—you may not find the support you need from your current network. Consider joining a support group to meet others who are dealing with similar challenges.
Improve your social skills.	If you feel awkward in social situations and just don't know what to say, try asking simple questions about the other person to get the ball rolling. If you're shy, it can be less intimidating to get to know others while doing shared activities—such as a bike ride or a knitting class—rather than just hanging out and talking. If you feel particularly anxious in social situations, consider talking to a therapist with experience in social anxiety and social-skills training.
Ask for help.	If you lack a strong support network and aren't sure where to start, there are resources you can turn to. Places of worship, senior and community centers, local libraries, refugee and immigrant groups, neighborhood health clinics, and local branches of national organizations such as Catholic Charities or the YMCA/YWCA may be able to help you identify services, support groups, and other programs in your community.

Source: American Psychological Association.

there is no substitute for face-to-face interactions. Try not to take support from family members for granted—saying "Thank you" now and then never hurts.

Building a strong social support network is a wise investment in one's overall physical and mental health, and you may live longer, too. However, it takes time to develop trusting relationships, so be patient, maintain a positive attitude, and try not to be discouraged. And remember that the process of creating a social support network should reduce the stress in your life, not add to it.

EXPERT COMMENTARY: SOCIAL ISOLATION AMONG OLDER ADULTS

Drug and alcohol problems that began during their younger years may worsen as people get older and as the difficulties of aging begin to multiply.

Yoko Sakuma Crume, Consultant
International Aging Practice and Policy

Dr. Crume is an international expert in aging societies, specializing in long-term-care issues and assistive technologies for older adults. She has a particular interest in aging in the urban environment because such a large and growing segment of the world's population lives in cities. Dr. Crume was formerly a social work professor at North Carolina A&T State University, and she now writes and lectures on global aging issues.

What do you see as the greatest issues regarding social isolation among older adults in urban areas, what are the major obstacles to addressing these issues, and what is your hope for the future?

You may be surprised to learn that many older adults living in the city are socially isolated, which means they have few social interactions even though they may live in the midst of a highly populated urban area, where social activities abound. How can this be? Our relationships change as we grow older, and we often lose contact with friends and work colleagues after retirement. Also, many older adults have mobility issues that prevent them from getting around (for example, going up and down steps or negotiating city curbs without assistance), and others suffer from poor health or audiovisual issues that makes socializing difficult. Some older adults choose to isolate themselves as they mourn the death of a loved one, perhaps a spouse of many years, and try to adjust to life without a close companion. And some older adults simply don't feel part of today's youth-oriented urban culture. The result is that a large number of older adults in urban areas live lonely and isolated lives.

To cope with their loneliness, some older adults turn to alcohol and drugs, and sadly, some decide to end their lives. In the United States, 14 percent of elderly emergency room admissions are the result of drug or alcohol problems, and older adults are hospitalized as often for alcohol-related abuse as for heart attacks. Additionally, because older adults often take multiple medicines that can interact with other drugs and alcohol, and because their physical strength and endurance are less than when they were younger, older adults often struggle to change bad habits and fight off addiction. Another health risk of alcohol drinking is the link with suicide. In the United States today, substance abuse disorder (especially drinking) is the second-most-common category of diagnosis among suicides involving the population age 65 and older.

As life expectancies increase, an increasing number of older adults experience debilitating and painful health and mental health conditions, including severe depression, that are often drivers of suicide.

As the population ages in the United States and worldwide, my hope is that we can be better about reaching out to older adults who live in social isolation in the city. Many cities have senior centers and other programs aimed at older adults, but too many remain at home and do not participate. Younger people can help by befriending their older neighbors, perhaps inviting them for dinner now and then or taking them out on errands. We also need to support organizations like the Village Movement, which is designed to help older adults live independently in the city by providing social activities, assistance with grocery shopping or getting to doctor appointments, and discount services making city living more affordable. There are also a number of volunteer ride services, where younger people assist older adults with their transportation needs. We need to help older adults understand the importance of social engagement as a way of avoiding social isolation, and we need to respect their right to pursue a fulfilling life, no matter how severe their disabilities. Let's all work together to solve this problem!

Solid Waste Management and Recycling

Cities across the world struggle with the management of waste because there is so much of it. For example, New York City generates an enormous volume of residential and institutional waste—over 12,000 tons per day throughout the year. Thanks to aggressive waste management and reduction programs instituted in a number of large metropolitan areas like New York City, the amount of waste generated in these urban areas is declining and waste recycling is increasing, resulting in less waste material going to municipal landfills and incinerators. Unfortunately, this is not the case for many other urban areas, particularly in developing nations, where waste amounts are on the upswing. Throughout the world, waste management represents one of the greatest challenges for urban areas, typically consuming 20 to 50 percent of the entire municipal operating budget.

Having an effective waste-management program in cities is important for several reasons, the most fundamental being public health. Urban wastes that are improperly managed can expose residents to disease, and the air pollution from trash collection and hauling trucks contributes to respiratory diseases and other health issues. Wastes disposed of in landfills create methane, a potent global warming gas, and incinerated wastes cause a variety of toxic air pollutants. On the other hand, when wastes are well managed and minimized, the environment benefits, city resources are conserved, and prices can fall on consumer goods that are recycled or reused.

Most waste-management issues in urban areas involve municipal solid waste (MSW). Definitions of MWS vary from country to country, but it is generally considered to include just about any type of waste generated by households, including paper, plastics, metal cans, and waste food. MSW also includes similar wastes from commercial, industrial, and institutional facilities, including schools and hospitals, and from public trash cans. Construction and demolition wastes (e.g., concrete, wallboard, wood, brick, and roofing materials) are often included in the MSW definition, as are waste materials from small workshops and cottage industries in developing countries. Due to their potential health risks, infectious medical and hazardous material wastes are ordinarily handled separately from MSW, often by private treatment and disposal facilities. Also, some medical facilities have their own incinerators for destroying potentially infectious wastes.

No matter how carefully a city regulates waste disposal, it is difficult for city waste managers to prevent some amount of hazardous material from contaminating their MSW. For example, residents cleaning up or renovating their homes may add to their household trash toxic paints and varnishes, pesticides, cleaning products, batteries, and used motor oil. Many cities in developed countries have been successful in minimizing this problem by encouraging residents to dispose of hazardous materials at special collection sites, where the materials may be neutralized, recycled, or disposed of at treatment and disposal facilities. Also, curbside recycling programs, where residents separate recyclable materials into special bins for collection by city workers, are increasingly common. However, in developing nations, waste-collection rules are less rigorous, and as a result, hazardous and nonhazardous waste materials are often mixed, sometimes causing toxic air pollution from landfills and contamination of groundwater.

Despite many successful municipal programs to reduce and recycle wastes, the overall amount of wastes generated in urban areas worldwide is growing. This phenomenon is due to increasing standards of living in many regions of the world, allowing people to buy more disposable items, often contained in throwaway packaging. As a result, there is an ongoing increase in the amount of waste per capita in urban areas, with high-income countries experiencing over the past few decades an average 3 percent rise per year in the quantity of waste generated. Also, cities are growing in size, especially in developing regions of the world, with increasing numbers of people moving into urban areas from surrounding rural areas, thereby swelling the volume of trash that cities must cope with.

The United States is one of the most wasteful countries on Earth. By some estimates, it produces up to a third of the world's solid wastes, while representing less than 5 percent of the global population. One reason for this anomaly is that people in the United States have grown accustomed to using items once and then tossing them away—the fate of about 80 percent of U.S. consumer-purchased items. Nearly half (by weight) of these items are packaging, containers, and paper or plastic products, such as paper bags and towels, plastic cups and plates, and shopping and trash bags. This one-use mindset is due, in part, to the low consumer cost of one-use items and the readily available land outside cities for landfill disposal. However, landfills convenient to cities are filling up, and as people become more conscious about environmental protection, many U.S. urban areas are embracing waste reduction and recycling programs, similar to steps already taken in many of the world's large metropolitan areas. A study by the Environmental Protection Agency (EPA) found that in 2016, the recycling industry created 757,000 jobs and $36.6 billion in wages, disproving the misconception that waste recycling is a drag on the economy.

The recycling and reuse of food wastes constitute a hot topic in many cities, where the sustainable management of wasted food products has been attracting much attention. The United Nations estimates that as much as one-third of all food produced for human consumption is wasted, and in the United States, where the average American throws away about a pound (a half-kilogram) of food every day, food wastes represent over 20 percent of all discarded MSW. Much of this is unsold food from grocery stores, unused food from restaurants, and discarded food from home refrigerators and pantries.

To address the food waste problem, the EPA has developed a hierarchy of actions for city managers and residents to follow. The elements of this hierarchy are listed here, arranged from top to lowest priority:

- **Source reduction**—reduce the volume of surplus food generated
- **Feed hungry people**—donate extra food to food banks, soup kitchens, and shelters
- **Feed animals**—divert food scraps to produce animal feed
- **Industrial uses**—provide waste oils for rendering and fuel conversion, and food scraps for anaerobic digestion to recovery energy
- **Composting**—create nutrient-rich soil amendment
- **Landfill/incineration**—use only as a last resort for disposal

The EPA believes that if cities implemented this hierarchy, the amount of waste food transported to MSW landfills and incinerators would be drastically reduced. One way that consumers and businesses can help achieve the first objective—reducing the surplus food volume—is to better understand the significance of expiration dates—the "best if used by," "best if used before," "sell by," and "use by" dates found on food packaging. Misconceptions abound regarding expiration dates, which are usually nothing more than manufacturers' best estimates about how long a food product will taste freshest. According to *Consumer Reports* (a U.S.-based, independent, nonprofit magazine that helps consumers make wise decisions about purchases), expiration dates are often conservative and may have little to do with how safe the food is. For example, nonperishable items like grains and dried and canned goods can often be used well past their expiration dates, although for meat, dairy, and eggs, the expiration dates are much more important. Many foods can be preserved beyond their expiration dates by refrigerating or freezing them. The U.S. Department of Agriculture created FoodKeeper, a computer and smartphone app that helps consumers determine how long foods are safe to eat based on the type of food, when the packaging was opened, and how long the food has been refrigerated or frozen.

In addition to reducing the amount of discarded food, consumers and businesses can cut back on the food waste sent to landfills and incinerators by composting their uneaten food. There are many types of food waste that are suitable for composting, including spoiled food, uneaten plate-scrapings, cooking oil and grease, and unused foods that remain after commercial food processing and packaging. In addition, huge amounts of food, disposed of by grocery stores because the expiration dates have passed or the food simply does not look as fresh as other food, could be composted or donated to food banks. Discarded food waste can also be kept out of municipal landfills and incinerators if sent to anaerobic digestion facilities, which may be stand-alone units or larger operations at farms or water resource recovery facilities. Anaerobic digestion involves a series of biological processes that break down food wastes and other organic material, giving off biogas (mostly methane and carbon dioxide) that can be captured and combusted to generate electricity and heat or processed into transportation fuel.

IMPACT ON URBAN HEALTH

Many nations have inadequate and unsustainable waste-management programs in their cities, including the sprawling urban areas in at least half of low-income countries that fail to meet even minimal standards for effective waste collection and management. These conditions lead to serious public health concerns as trash accumulates on streets and in local dumps, providing conditions conducive for the propagation of rodents and insects that can spread viral and parasitic diseases. Many slum areas in these countries have grown up in the vicinity of landfills, where infectious diseases are rampant. A related problem involves inadequate sanitation infrastructure, where human excreta and toilet paper may be mixed with municipal wastes. In many cities, even in industrialized countries, residents sometimes burn waste materials in the open or in drums, resulting in a toxic mix of air pollutants. (Although this practice is often banned, enforcement is seldom rigorous.)

Children are particularly susceptible to diseases associated with improperly managed and disposed of urban wastes. Uncollected waste piles can be infested with vermin like rats and become ideal breeding environments for disease-carrying mosquitoes. As children play outside, they are more likely than adults to come into contact with wastes and develop an illness. Additionally, children's bodies are more susceptible to disease because their metabolic pathways for detoxifying foreign agents are not fully developed and because they ingest more food and water and inhale more air per unit body weight, leading to higher levels of exposure to toxic and infectious agents.

Workers who collect and transport MSW are also at increased risk of disease and injury, particularly in developing countries, where the risk of infections and parasites among MSW workers is 3 to 6 times higher than the general population and the risk of diarrhea is 10 times higher. If hazardous wastes are present, MSW workers face an increased risk of serious, life-threatening illnesses, including cancer, organ failure, and metabolic dysfunction, and there is also an increased risk of birth defects. Also, puncture wounds caused by pieces of glass, needles, and other sharp objects are very common, leading to infections, tetanus, hepatitis, and HIV exposure. In this regard, wearing protective equipment—face masks, gloves, steel boots, long-sleeve shirts, and long pants—is especially important. MSW workers often experience extreme weather conditions and lift heavy objects, increasing their risk of severe heat and cold exposure, dehydration, and physical injury, and they also may suffer from hearing loss caused by loud machinery.

In slum areas, waste-picking, a common profession among the poorest members of society, is often an important part of the city's informal recycling infrastructure. Items picked up at landfills and dump sites can be sold, providing some amount of income (even if meager) for families living in poverty, and the poorest families may even search for discarded food products. Waste-pickers work under highly unhygienic and unsafe conditions, risking illness and accidents on a daily basis, as they roam over piles of spoiled food, broken bottles, and demolition debris. Thus, it is no surprise that these individuals suffer high rates of infectious diseases, bronchitis, asthma, anemia, and conjunctivitis—illnesses that are always more common among the young waste-pickers.

The ultimate solution to waste-picking, of course, is to eliminate poverty. But given that this is unlikely to happen anytime soon, another approach has been to provide safety equipment, such as protective gloves and boots. Sadly, many of these desperate people opt to sell these items to buy food for their families instead of keeping them for themselves. In some locations, health workers provide vaccination programs and locate health facilities near landfills and dump sites, and city officials work to reduce child labor and provide schooling for children.

WHAT CITIES ARE DOING ABOUT WASTE MANAGEMENT AND RECYCLING

Cities in developing parts of the world have a variety of waste-collection and -disposal strategies, ranging from local waste dumps and the open burning of trash to sophisticated landfilling and incineration systems. Within industrialized countries, waste management often involves a complex array of options, including curbside trash pickup, hauling to a landfill or incinerator, recycling programs, waste reduction and reuse initiatives, and city ordinances aimed at reducing waste at commercial businesses and construction sites. Also, some cities have developed visionary "zero-waste" plans, with the goal of eliminating waste taken to landfills or incinerators through aggressive recycling and reuse programs.

One of the world's most ambitious zero-waste plans can be found in New York City, where city officials want to reduce by 90 percent the amount of waste material that it sends to landfills by 2030. Through a combination of waste reduction, reuse, recycling, composting, and anaerobic digestion programs, New York is diverting large quantities of waste from landfills and reducing the number of trash trucks on city streets, thereby relieving traffic congestion and reducing air pollution emissions as well as cutting back on waste. The city's waste-reduction program has a long way to go to achieve its goal, but eventually, the city hopes to save more than $310 million per year in fuel and other transportation costs associated with waste collection and transportation. Additionally, the reduced traffic and air pollution will be good for pedestrian safety and health, leading to a better quality of life for many residents.

San Francisco is another city with ambitious goals for reducing wastes that require disposal. The city has committed to following a waste-management hierarchy wherein waste prevention comes first, followed by waste reduction and reuse, recycling, and finally composting of organic wastes. City leaders believe that by making San Francisco a zero-waste city, they will be protecting the environment; reducing greenhouse gases (GHGs), such as methane from landfills; and creating jobs in waste-management industries like recycling. Already, San Francisco has become the top city in North America for recycling and food scrap composting, it sends less trash to landfills than any other major U.S. city, and it has decreased the disposal of plastic bags by 100 million per year. Key to San Francisco's success is citizen engagement, where many residents enthusiastically support and participate in the city's waste-management programs. Also, the city has stringent recycling requirements for both residents and businesses, and it was the first city in the United States to pass a mandatory composting law.

Many other cities also have aggressive waste-management programs. For example, in Toronto, the trash collection fleet runs on compressed natural gas to reduce air pollution, the city has two anaerobic digestion facilities for organic wastes, and its curbside collection program includes a special bin for most types of food waste (i.e., bread, cake, candy, cereals, cookies, dairy products, eggs and shells, fish products, fruits, meat, nuts, pasta, poultry, rice, and vegetables). Seattle requires that construction and demolition contractors collect recyclable materials on site, and the city uses a sophisticated computer system to optimize their waste-collection and -management systems. And Arlington, Virginia, a densely populated area near Washington, D.C., with about half its residents living in condominiums and apartment buildings, has established regulations for managing waste at these multifamily facilities, and waste movement is tracked with radio-transmitting identification tags on collection carts.

In Europe, nearly 400 cities have committed to working toward zero waste by joining Zero Waste Europe, an organization that supports a network of 29 national and local nongovernmental organizations promoting a zero-waste strategy as a way to make Europe more sustainable. A multitude of waste-management approaches are used by these cities, such as minimizing food waste, reducing product packaging for products sold in the city (or requiring that the packaging be recyclable or compostable), separating recyclable items at homes or neighborhood collection points, and partnering with local organizations promoting the reuse of waste materials. Some European municipalities have already achieved impressive recycling rates of 80 to 90 percent of all recyclable wastes. Several success stories include (1) Italian officials calling on coffee chain stores to stop using disposable cups and glasses; (2) restaurants offering reusable lunchboxes at more than 400 restaurants in Switzerland and Germany; (3) waste recycling, reuse, and reduction programs being introduced in Madrid, allowing the city to shut down its municipal waste incinerator by 2025; and (4) the Hotel Ribno in Bled, Slovenia, becoming the country's first zero-waste hotel by engaging both employees and guests in waste-reduction habits and practices.

RECOMMENDATIONS FOR CITY DWELLERS

The most effective approach for reducing waste is not to create it in the first place. Along with reuse and recycling, these are the easiest ways for individuals living in the city to contribute to waste management in their neighborhoods. Some examples include the following:

- Learn about voluntary and mandatory recycling programs in the community and divert recyclable trash into recycling bins.
- Buy used items, such as clothing and building materials, which are often just as good as new items—and cheaper too.
- Purchase items where the manufacturer has incorporated less packaging or packaging that can be recycled or composted, and avoid items packaged in materials that end up in the trash. Sometimes buying in bulk can reduce packaging while saving money, provided you really need the items and can use them in a reasonable time frame (e.g., before food goes bad).
- When shopping, always give preference to reusable over disposable items. For example, take your own cup or thermos bottle to a coffee shop, and when purchasing takeout meals, bring along your own silverware rather than using plastic eating utensils.
- Repair clothing, appliances, automobile tires, and other products so that they do not have to be thrown away and replaced.
- Rather than buying new items, consider borrowing or renting items that you will use infrequently or only once.

Another way to reduce waste is to make donations to local churches, thrift stores, schools, and other nonprofit organizations dedicated to helping people in need. There is often high demand for clothing, appliances, furniture, tools, and books. You will feel good about helping others, and you may be able to take a charitable deduction on your income tax, to boot.

CITY SPOTLIGHT: TORONTO—GREEN LIVING MADE EASY AND FUN

Recognizing that a healthy environment and healthy lifestyle go hand in hand, this large metropolitan area has engaged thousands of citizens in activities aimed at cleaning up the environment, reducing waste, and eating healthy foods. (And there is even a program to protect the bees.)

Toronto, one of the most diverse urban areas in the world, is a center of higher education and home to a thriving international business community. As Canada's largest city, Toronto is also focused on becoming "clean, green, and sustainable" through numerous initiatives aimed at reducing GHG emissions, improving air and water quality, reducing solid-waste generation, expanding public transportation systems, developing renewable energy, and establishing vibrant green spaces. That is a lot to take on, but steady progress has been made, and the city was recently invited to join 100 Resilient Cities, a global network of cities demonstrating a commitment to building resilience to the physical, social, and economic challenges that are a growing part of the twenty-first century.

To help achieve its sustainability goals, the city formed Live Green Toronto, a multifaceted program that helps residents and businesses live and work in environmentally sustainable ways, with the ultimate aim of becoming a healthier and more resilient city. The program provides tools and resources for building a sustainable community, and it sponsors many public events throughout the year, including over 100 festivals, trade shows, and workshops. By creating fun and convenient opportunities for people throughout the city, Live Green Toronto is helping residents enjoy a healthy lifestyle by being active, eating locally grown foods, and living in a clean environment.

Among the many programs recently sponsored by Live Green Toronto are (1) Community Environment Days, an annual event making it easy to donate electronics and other items for reuse or recycling, dispose of hazardous household wastes, and pick up free compost; (2) Blue Water Day, an event raising awareness about protecting local water resources; (3) Clean Toronto Together, an annual spring cleanup engaging nearly 200,000 community participants at over 1,000 local cleanup events, and (4) Local Food Fest, an occasion celebrating the city's diverse food culture, outstanding chefs, and locally grown foods. Toronto's Live Green Card promotes the purchase of ecofriendly products and services by providing discounts at hundreds of participating businesses, and the Live Green smartphone app makes shopping for green products and services easier.

Grants and loans are also available to individuals, community groups, and commercial businesses for a variety of projects related to energy conservation, environmental protection, and climate change, such as installing energy-efficient windows, upgrading appliances and heating/air conditioning units, and reducing waste. Grants are even available for installing green roofs (waterproof roofing covered with soil for vegetation, such as grass, shrubs, and gardens) and cool roofs (light-colored roofing that reflects sunlight away from buildings, keeping them cooler in the summer). Both techniques are components of the city's plan to reduce GHGs.

With support from the Live Green Toronto program, the city recently became Canada's first "bee city," a nationwide program to protect the native bee and honeybee populations that have been declining in Canada and the United States. Toronto's bee-city resolution notes that globally, about 85 percent of flowering plants depend on insect pollinators, and in Canada, one of every three bites of food is courtesy of bees and other pollinating insects. Toronto's strategy for protecting bees includes establishing pollinator-friendly habitats across the city, engaging local communities in planting native species, teaching children about the importance of bees, supporting a local butterfly trail, and running a Horticulture School of Excellence to instruct city staff about pollinator-friendly plantings, including native plants in city parks. Toronto has also banned the use of pesticides suspected of killing bees.

A key to Live Green Toronto's success is in mobilizing well over 1,000 volunteers who are trained in a variety of environmental and lifestyle topics, including waste management, sustainable transportation, climate change, green buildings, urban forestry, local foods, and food waste. (The city wants to cut back on food waste, with the goal of averaging no more than about US$1,200 lost to such waste annually per single-family household.) Volunteers sponsor or attend local events, educate the public on environmental sustainability, and participate in neighborhood projects. Social media is widely used to promote events, and to reach out to all segments of Toronto's diverse population, the volunteers collectively speak over 70 different languages.

Measuring the success of a program like Live Green Toronto is difficult because it touches lives in so many different ways. However, if nothing else, the program appears to have been highly successful in raising awareness about urban environmental and sustainability issues, including the importance of a clean and green city to good health, and it has inspired thousands of city residents to get involved with community projects aimed at reducing waste, greening their homes and businesses, and eating more locally grown food.

Stress Management

We all have stress in our lives, but this is especially true for urban dwellers, who must contend with a variety of stressful situations common to city life. Mental health experts tell us that some stress is normal, and even good when it helps us develop the skills needed to handle difficult situations. However, when stress builds up to a point where it disrupts our daily activities, interferes with work or school, or leads to depression, it is time to do something about it. Recognizing stress and learning how to cope with it are important talents that everyone needs to develop.

Stress, a condition characterized by emotional or physical tension, is a reaction to a situation that is threatening or otherwise causes feelings of anxiety. Stress can result from a traumatic event, such as an automobile accident, loss of a job, or death of a loved one. Happy events can also cause stress, like planning a wedding or preparing a big holiday meal. We often describe sources of stress in terms of "macrostressors," which encompass major life events, and "microstressors," which are the smaller stresses that we experience while going about our daily routines—getting to work on time, preparing for an exam in school, or being stuck in traffic are examples. While coping with macrostressors can be very challenging, it is actually the buildup of microstressors, day after day, that can have the most devastating effect on our health and well-being, wearing us down and affecting our self-worth and confidence.

Stress need not always be viewed in a negative light. For many people, learning how to cope with stress helps develop skills and competencies, such as someone who finds public speaking stressful but learns to overcome these emotions through practice and experience. People who are most successful in life are often those who see stressful situations as opportunities for personal growth, whereas people who avoid stress may miss out on these opportunities. However, when stress builds up from a traumatic event or a series of daily stressors, even the most self-confident people can feel anxiety and self-doubt. When this occurs, it may be time to slow down, relax with family and friends, and consider professional counseling.

People who live or work in busy urban areas are often subject to an onslaught of microstressors, such as driving in heavy traffic, riding in crowded subway cars, and rushing to get to work or school on time. City noises and flashing neon signs can also bring on stress, as can neighborhood crime and pollution. The loneliness caused by social isolation is another form of stress increasingly common in urban areas. This is surprising, given that most large cities are densely populated, where there are people almost everywhere you look. But many city people, particularly older adults, and others with limited mobility, live alone and have few opportunities for social activities. Younger residents also can suffer from social isolation if they work long hours, leaving little time for relaxation with friends. For socially isolated people, the city can be a lonely and stressful place.

Stress can also build up from societal concerns, particularly those issues which we hear about almost daily in the news media and which we may feel we have little control over. For example, because of our political leanings or religious beliefs, we may have very strong emotions about certain issues that others feel differently about, and trying to understand and accept other viewpoints can be frustrating and stressful. Also, people may be upset over the perceived slow pace of governmental action on issues that some may view as crises.

Table 25 summarizes a recent American Psychological Association survey on what specific societal concerns cause Americans stress when thinking about the state of the nation. Healthcare and the economy are high on the list of these stressful issues, but other concerns like trust in government and crime are relatively close behind. The survey found that millennials (people born in the 1980s or 1990s) had the highest reported stress levels, but the greatest increase in stress from earlier surveys was reported among older adults. Women, on average, reported greater stress levels than men, and there were also variations by race, ethnicity, and age. About 95 percent of American adults say that they follow the news regularly, and 56 percent say doing so causes them stress.

Table 25   Causes of Stress When Thinking About the Nation

Issue	Percent Feeling Stress Over the Issue
Healthcare	43
Economy	35
Trust in government	32
Crime	31
Hate crimes	31
Wars/conflicts with other countries	30
Terrorist attacks in the United States	30
High taxes	28
Social security	26
Government controversies and scandals	25
Unemployment and low wages	22
Climate change and environmental issues	21

Source: American Psychological Association.

How do people know when they are experiencing stress? Here are some signs to look for:

- anxiety about the future
- difficulty concentrating and making decisions
- feeling guilty about situations, even if beyond your control
- frequent crying, anger, sadness, or irritability
- frustration and feeling helpless
- headaches, aches and pains, upset stomach, or loss of appetite
- increased alcohol consumption, drug use, or smoking
- loss of interest in daily activities and wanting to be alone
- nightmares, problems sleeping at night, or sleeping too much
- shortness of breath, elevated blood pressure, or heart palpitations

Strong emotions brought on by stress, such as feeling sad, anxious, or angry, are natural—we all have strong emotions from time to time, and they are usually temporary, lasting just a few hours or days. But when our emotions last longer, they can take over our lives and interfere with our daily activities and relationships. When this happens, depression may set in, some people may turn to alcohol or drugs, and others may become habitual cigarette smokers. When stress becomes too great, school and job performance may suffer, positive relationships may end, and sadly, a few people may take their own lives.

When assessing stress within a city, experts often look to population density as a key factor. As the number of people living and working in close proximity increases, noise and pollution become more bothersome, exposure to infectious diseases occurs with greater frequency, and people suffer more from stress-related illnesses. This is especially concerning in parts of Asia, Africa, South America, and the Middle East, where some of the world's most densely populated cities can be found—Bogota, Colombia; Jakarta, Indonesia; Karachi, Pakistan; Lagos, Nigeria; Manila, the Philippines; Mumbai, India; and Tehran, Iran, particularly stand out for their population densities and stressful circumstances for many inhabitants. The worst areas are the slums surrounding these and other megacities, where extreme poverty forces many people to live in single-room shacks, often inhabited by a number of family members. On the other hand, while cities like London, New York City, and Tokyo and the city-state of Singapore also have high population densities, the relative wealth of these cities has resulted in highly efficient infrastructure and decent wages that help make city life tolerable, if not enjoyable, for many residents. The more affluent residents of these cities may live in luxury high-rises, where the surrounding population density has little bearing on the quality of life. (For more information on population density, see the "Population Growth and Overcrowding" entry.)

IMPACT ON URBAN HEALTH

Today, more than half the world's population lives in cities, and urban population is expected to climb to over two-thirds by 2050. As more people become city dwellers, it is increasingly important that health professionals understand the symptoms of stress associated with city life and the ways that stress can affect public health.

It is not surprising that people living in densely populated and congested urban areas become irritable and anxious from time to time. Squeezing into a packed subway train or getting stuck in a traffic jam would wear on anyone's nerves. However, a number of research studies have demonstrated that people born and raised in cities also experience more serious stress-related problems, such as higher rates of psychosis, anxiety disorders, and depression. Additionally, other studies have found an association between schizophrenia and urban living. There are various factors that probably contribute to these mental health conditions, including heredity, socioeconomic status, substance abuse, childhood exposure to the urban environment, and possibly a tendency for people predisposed to mental illness to move to the city. Nevertheless, many health professionals believe that the added stresses encountered by city residents contribute to these disorders. One theory is that in a busy and congested urban area, the constant sensory input to the human brain can overwhelm the parts of the brain involved with regulating emotional responses and managing stress.

Children and teens living in the city are at increased risk of developing posttraumatic stress disorder (PTSD) if they have experienced sexual or physical abuse, violent crime, family violence, bullying, the injury or death of a loved one, a school shooting, or some other traumatic event. PTSD is an intense physical and emotional response to a traumatic event that may last for weeks or months, and it is a common affliction of military personnel returning from battle zones. Symptoms include (1) reliving the event (e.g., flashbacks, nightmares, and emotional responses to reminders of the event); (2) avoiding places and activities associated with the event; and (3) increased arousal (e.g., being overly alert or easily startled). PTSD may cause panic attacks, depression, drug abuse, and suicidal thoughts. For young children, PTSD may be apparent in their play (e.g., they may act out part of the trauma).

While stress is a major concern of urban areas, cities typically offer a rich cultural environment that sometimes can reduce stress and improve the quality of life for many residents. Having more educational and entertainment opportunities, as well as better healthcare options and a higher overall standard of living, makes for a more relaxed and healthier lifestyle. Many city residents manage their stress by attending a concert, ball game, or lecture, or by enjoying a meal at a fine restaurant—opportunities that may be missing from more rural settings. These more enjoyable aspects of city life may be protective factors against stress for those residents who have sufficient leisure time and financial resources to take advantage of them.

WHAT CITIES ARE DOING ABOUT STRESS MANAGEMENT

City planners have long recognized that urban design—the accumulation and arrangement of buildings, roadways, shopping areas, and green spaces—has a strong influence on our mental outlook and happiness.

Streetscapes made up of a mixture of small shops and restaurants, shade trees, and benches for resting are conducive to walking at a slow pace and striking up friendly conversations with strangers, and stress and mental fatigue can be further reduced by spending time in nearby parks, community gardens, and other green spaces. On the other hand, when people encounter the stark facade of a modern high-rise building—often glass, brick, or stone spanning an entire city block—they pick up their pace and rush to their destination, leaving no opportunity for a relaxing walk or conversation. To improve city life and reduce stress, a goal of many urban planners is to encourage pedestrian-friendly streetscapes, green areas, and mixed-use high-rise developments incorporating street-level shopping and landscaping.

A related city-planning objective is to concentrate jobs, residences, shops, schools, and parks in several decentralized areas around town (e.g., near subway stations), allowing residents to reach their destinations by walking or taking a short bus ride. This approach to urban planning helps reduce stress by minimizing commuting time, improving traffic flow, and helping city residents include physical exercise (e.g., walking to school or work) in their daily routine. To further improve the quality of life in the city, architects are increasingly incorporating greenery into new buildings (e.g., indoor gardens or walls covered with vines). Exterior landscaping has been improving too, and many new buildings feature green roofs, where occupants can tend a garden, get some fresh air, and take in a spectacular view of the city.

Another important goal of modern urban design is to create opportunities for social connections. Health professionals have observed that when social activities are missing from someone's life, stress and unhappiness build up, leading to a greater risk of antisocial behavior and illness. To encourage social connections, urban planners are expanding the number of parks and other green areas where people can meet, sponsoring farmers' markets and street fairs, and designing shopping areas that are conducive to social interaction. Social connections are particularly important for older adults, many living alone in the city and suffering from social isolation.

Most large cities offer mental health services to help residents cope with chronic stress, anxiety, depression, and other mental health conditions. Some examples of these services are:

- addiction counseling
- anger management
- clinical services for those without insurance

- crisis intervention and hotlines
- educational and preventive-care services
- individual and family therapy
- individualized treatment planning
- medication monitoring
- psychiatric assessment and treatment
- psychosocial rehabilitation
- referrals to care providers and agencies

City governments are helping their own employees handle stress by providing programs that balance work and family life, such as flexible working hours, opportunities to work remotely (e.g., at home), and maternity and paternity leave. Many companies have also adopted these policies, and some firms go even further by providing free snack foods and gourmet coffee, gym and workout facilities, exercise and weight-loss incentives, health clinics and meditation rooms, on-call massage therapists, gripe sessions to air complaints, and group social outings. Some companies limit after-hours emails and encourage full use of vacation time, and a few firms even allow employees to bring their pets to work. These and other benefits help manage stress while improving productivity (e.g., fewer missed workdays due to illness), increasing employee retention, and cutting healthcare costs.

RECOMMENDATIONS FOR URBAN DWELLERS

Managing stress is an important skill that we all need to learn. Regardless of age and circumstances, there are several important steps to preventing stress from overtaking our lives.

First, be connected socially. This means being in the habit of spending time regularly with family and friends and feeling free to share with them your joys and concerns. Knowing that others care about you and are willing to help with your problems, just as you are willing to help them, goes a long way in relieving stress and living a healthy life. Also, develop personal relationships with a counselor, member of the clergy, and health professionals whom you can turn to for advice when problems arise.

Next, plan fun events and other activities to help you relax and avoid taking life too seriously. By being active in social events involving friends and family, you can relieve stress and enjoy life more. For some people, volunteer work can be very therapeutic by taking your mind off your own problems and focusing on the needs of others. Sometimes sitting in the park or taking a walk on a nice day can help you refocus, too.

Avoid turning to alcohol and drugs as a remedy for your troubles because in the long run, they will only add to your problems and increase your level of stress. Some people can tolerate light or moderate alcohol consumption, and some doctors even suggest a little wine for relaxation and improved sleep. However, never increase alcohol consumption to help cope with chronic stress and depression because doing so can actually make matters worse. And you also risk alcohol dependency and becoming a binge drinker.

Finally, to manage stress, it is very important to take good care of yourself—eat well, get plenty of sleep, and exercise regularly. By adopting a heathy lifestyle, you can undo unhealthy habits that lead to stress and feel better about taking control of your life. Avoid taking on too many responsibilities, and set aside personal time every day for relaxation—listening to music, reading a book, or watching a comedy on television.

Sometimes you may feel stress and anxiety even if you are doing all the right things to relieve stress and stay healthy. For example, perhaps there has been a death in your family or you are not getting along with your boss at work. Or, maybe you are experiencing stressful feelings for no clear reason other than you are too busy and not relaxing enough. The Centers for Disease Control and Prevention (CDC) advises that you may need help from a licensed mental health professional, doctor, or community or faith-based organization if you (1) have symptoms of stress, like feeling sad or depressed, for more than two weeks; (2) are unable to take care of yourself or your family; (3) are unable to do your job or go to school because of your stress; (3) are using alcohol or drugs because of stress; or (4) are thinking about suicide. If you experience any of these symptoms, you need to seek professional help right away. Consider reaching out to your mental health provider, your primary doctor or other healthcare provider, a close friend or loved one, or someone in your faith community. Also, the CDC and other national and local organizations provide excellent resources for dealing with stress, anxiety, and depression, including crisis intervention centers and hotlines. In the United States, the National Suicide Prevention Lifeline is 800-273-TALK (800-273-8255), and you can chat online at https://suicidepreventionlifeline.org.

Walkable and Bike-Friendly Neighborhoods

A neighborhood is "walkable" when a person in reasonably good health can walk to nearby destinations without difficulty, such as a grocery store, doctor's office, or park. The requirements for being "bike-friendly" are a little different—the city must provide bicycle lanes, pathways, and other infrastructure that allows bicyclists to make reasonably steady progress, such as commuting to work across town, without endangering themselves or others. Walkable and bike-friendly neighborhoods are good for health, and they also help cities reduce traffic congestion and pollution.

Urban planners have long recognized that people enjoy living in communities where they can walk or ride a bicycle to destinations rather than fighting the city traffic. People who routinely walk and ride bicycles are generally healthier than those who do not, and they suffer lower levels of stress. This helps explain why so many people in walkable cities like New York City and San Francisco have given up their automobiles in favor in walking and bicycling. No one enjoys the frustration of negotiating busy city streets in their cars and searching for parking spots, and in many big cities, automobile excise taxes, insurance, and parking fees can be quite expensive. Of course, not all cities and neighborhoods are conducive to walking and bicycling—most are not—and driving a car is more of a necessity.

How do cities become walkable and bike-friendly? Much has to do with the layout and design of a city—decisions likely make many years ago. If sidewalks are missing from neighborhoods, if roads lack bicycle lanes, and if destinations are far apart, cities have an uphill battle in becoming walkable and bike-friendly. Nevertheless, many urban areas have made remarkable progress in recent years in accommodating bicycle traffic and in designing local communities where homes, offices, commercial businesses, schools, and houses of worship are within a convenient walking distance from each other. A study by CEOs for Cities, a nonprofit organization promoting collaboration among urban leaders, found that houses in walkable communities command a higher sale price, concluding that "the property value premium for walkability seems to be higher in more populous urban areas and those with extensive transit, suggesting that the value gains associated with walkability are greatest when people have real alternatives to living without an automobile."

To help assess and improve the walkability of cities, a walk score is often calculated using the Walk Score website (walkscore.com). A walk score is a number between 0 and 100 that measures the walkability of a city or any address, neighborhood, or ZIP code within the city, based on an analysis of walking routes to nearby amenities and pedestrian friendliness, taking into account population density and various road metrics. The Walk Score website also provides several other scoring systems, including a bike score, which is based on an analysis of infrastructure, hills, destinations, road connectivity, and number of bike commuters. Tables 26 and 27 describe the walk score and bike score ranking systems.

Using the Walk Score methodology, the top 10 walkable large cities in the United States, and their walkability scores, are:

1. New York (89.2)
2. San Francisco (86.0)
3. Boston (80.9)
4. Miami (79.2)
5. Philadelphia (79.0)
6. Chicago (77.8)
7. Washington, D.C. (77.3)
8. Seattle (73.1)
9. Oakland (72.0)
10. Long Beach, California (69.9)

It may be surprising to see that a big, congested city like New York ranks first in walkability, but just about every neighborhood in this city is walkable, and residents are seldom farther than a 10- to 15-minute walk from a

Table 26   Walk Score Ranking System

Score	Description
90–100	**Walker's Paradise**—daily errands do not require a car
70–89	**Very Walkable**—most errands can be accomplished on foot
50–69	**Somewhat Walkable**—some errands can be accomplished on foot
25–49	**Car-Dependent**—most errands require a car
0–24	**Car-Dependent**—almost all errands require a car

Source: Walk Score, Inc.

Table 27   Bike Score Ranking System

Score	Bike Score Description
90–100	**Biker's Paradise**—daily errands can be accomplished on a bike
70–89	**Very Bikeable**—biking is convenient for most trips
50–69	**Bikeable**—some bike infrastructure
0–49	**Somewhat Bikeable**—minimal bike infrastructure

Source: Walk Score, Inc.

subway station. There are also bike-share programs and miles of bike lanes, making access to the city's museums, restaurants, and parks easy. As a consequence, many New York residents have lived their entire lives without owning a car. However, the walk scores for New York and the other top 10 cities are outliers—most large cities have much lower scores. The average walk score for the 100 largest U.S. cities is just 48, corresponding to a city classification of "car-dependent."

The top 10 cities for bicycling look a little different from the top 10 walkable cities. Here is the list:

1. Minneapolis (81.9)
2. Portland (81.2)
3. Chicago (71.5)
4. Denver (71.3)

5. San Francisco (70.7)

6. Seattle (70.0)

7. Boston (69.0)

8. New York (67.7)

9. Washington, D.C. (66.9)

10. Sacramento (65.9)

Minneapolis scores highest, in part, because of its Nice Ride bicycle-rental program, which makes available over 3,000 bicycles at more than 400 stations across the city. Also, the city has an extensive network of paths and off-road cycling trails connecting a number of parklands. Livability is further enhanced by the city's excellent system of buses, light rail, and commuter rail.

Notice that San Francisco is among the top five cities on both the walk and bike lists. Its streets and neighborhoods are very walkable, and ready access to the bus, rail, and subway systems allows residents to travel throughout the city with relative ease. Bicycling has become a very attractive transportation option for many San Francisco residents due to the limited supply and high cost of parking spaces and the frequent traffic congestion. And the charming cable cars and marvelous views of the bay are added bonuses of living in walkable and bike-friendly San Francisco.

As with the walk scores, the bike scores for Minneapolis, San Francisco, and the other top 10 cities are outliers, with most large cities having much lower scores. The average bike score for the 100 largest U.S. cities is just 49, a score corresponding to a city classification of "somewhat bikeable."

In addition to the health and environmental benefits of walking and bicycling, many big city urbanites take pride in learning to get by without an automobile, thereby saving the expenses and headaches that come with owning a car. The Automobile Association of America (AAA) estimates that the average cost to own and operate a car in the United States is around $8,850, a figure that includes costs for fuel, maintenance, repairs, insurance, license and registration taxes, depreciation, and loan interest for a car driven an average 15,000 miles (24,140 kilometers) per year. There are expenses associated with walking and bicycling too (e.g., the costs of walking shoes, rain gear, and a bicycle), but these expenses are insignificant by comparison. Even when owning a car, expenses can be cut by walking or bicycling to destinations that are nearby. For example, 21 percent of vehicle trips are 1 mile (1.6 kilometers) or less, and 46 percent are 3 miles (4.8 kilometers) or less—distances easily traversed by walking or bicycling. Over a quarter of all vehicle trips are for running errands like shopping and for eating out, activities that could easily be accomplished in a walkable neighborhood.

Healthy communities having opportunities for exercise and physical activity are often economically strong communities. In recent testimony before the U.S. Senate's Committee on Health, Education, Labor, and Pensions, the surgeon general of the United States, Vice Admiral Jerome M. Adams, explained it this way: "The health and economy of communities are often strongly correlated. Healthier communities tend to be economically more prosperous, and vice versa. Improved community conditions for health, such as clean and safe neighborhoods, access to healthful food options, and opportunities for exercise and physical activity, can help positively influence health behaviors and lead to a more productive workforce."

IMPACT ON URBAN HEALTH

Public health professionals recognized years ago that exercise, whether consisting of walking, bicycling, or working out at the gym, has a strong beneficial effect on health. For children, these benefits include developing healthy musculoskeletal tissues (i.e., bones, muscles, and joints) and a healthy cardiovascular system, improving coordination and movement control, and maintaining healthy body weight. Additionally, physical activity can improve symptoms of anxiety and depression, help social development by providing opportunities for self-expression, build self-confidence, and improve social interaction. There is also some evidence that physical activity among younger people may help them adopt other healthy behaviors, such as avoiding tobacco, alcohol, and drugs, and performance in school may also improve.

Adults also experience health improvements when they take advantage of exercise opportunities in their communities. Generally, adults who are more active have lower rates of coronary heart disease, high blood pressure, stroke, type 2 diabetes, metabolic syndrome, colon and breast cancer, depression, and mortality from all causes. Also, they are less likely to have a hip or vertebral fracture, and they are more likely to have a healthy body mass index. Older adults experience similar benefits of physical activity; plus they are less likely than their peers who do not exercise to experience a fall and to have impaired cognitive functions and other functional and role limitations.

Some research suggests that walkable environments encourage more creativity and healthy social interactions, and there may be a connection between walkability and reduced crime resulting from having more people on the street to observe potential criminal activity, hence deterring it. A less direct, but no less important, impact of walkable and bike-friendly neighborhoods is that as people depend less on automobiles, air pollution and greenhouse gas emissions from these motor vehicles are reduced. Fewer automobiles on the streets also means there are fewer opportunities for people to be injured in an automobile accident or struck by a car when crossing a street. When cities incorporate traffic safety measures to protect pedestrians and bicyclists, such as traffic-calming islands, well-marked street crossings, and bike lanes, research demonstrates that the risk of injuries and fatalities is significantly reduced.

By reducing vehicle speeds in walkable and bike-friendly neighborhoods, city planners have observed a significant reduction in pedestrian injuries. Pedestrians suffer more serious injuries when struck by high-speed vehicles, and many accidents involving pedestrians would be prevented entirely if the vehicle been traveling more slowly, giving the driver and pedestrian more time to react. According to the AAA, the average risk of severe injury for a pedestrian struck by a vehicle is 10 percent at an impact speed of 16 miles per hour (25.7 kilometers per hour), and this increases to 90 percent at 46 miles per hour (74.0 kilometers per hour). Similarly, the risk of death is 10 percent at an impact speed of 23 miles per hour (37.0 kilometers per hour), increasing to 90 percent at 58 miles per hour (93.3 kilometers per hour). (These risks are somewhat higher for older adults.) Of course, changing speed limits does not automatically translate into slower speeds and fewer injuries and deaths—good signage, traffic enforcement, and street design are also required. For example, regardless of the speed limit, for every 3 feet (0.9 meter) a street is narrowed, cars travel about 9 miles per hour (14.5 kilometers per hour) slower.

WHAT CITIES ARE DOING ABOUT WALKABLE AND BIKE-FRIENDLY NEIGHBORHOODS

Despite extensive literature and experience, city planners continue to struggle with what makes a city walkable and bike-friendly, a goal that is not nearly as easy as it may seem. There are some cities that have many walking and bicycling amenities, including sidewalks, bicycle paths and lanes, and parks, and yet, few people are seen taking advantage of these amenities. On the other hand, some cities largely lacking these amenities are observed to be full of walkers and bicyclists. To be sure, these amenities are critical, but other factors are also at play, such as the presence of narrow streets in business districts where the traffic slows down, visually attractive roadside businesses that are welcoming to everyone, benches and other informal gathering spots, local government support, and community pride and a commitment to making neighborhoods better places to live. Some research suggests that communities that include recent immigrants can be particularly vibrant, as the newcomers introduce culturally interesting foods and customs while embracing the neighborhood's walkability. Tables 28 and 29 list the attributes that many city planners consider when designing walk- and bike-friendly communities.

In designing a walkable community, city planners often take into account the distance that urban dwellers are willing to walk. In the United States,

Table 28   Basics of a Walk-Friendly Community

- The walking environment should be easy to use and understand.
- The walking environment should seamlessly connect people to places. It should be continuous, with complete sidewalks and well-designed curb ramps and street crossings.
- Pedestrian and driver sight distances should be maintained near driveways and intersections.
- Pedestrians must be able to cross roads safely. Municipalities have an obligation to provide safe and convenient crossing opportunities.
- The safety of all street users, particularly more vulnerable groups (e.g., children, older adults, and people with disabilities) must be considered when designing streets.
- Uncontrolled crossings on narrow streets with low volumes and speeds should be allowed. In these locations, provide marked crosswalks, pedestrian crossing signs, and regulatory signs that indicate a yield requirement to pedestrians on the part of drivers.
- Active control crossings for all wide streets with high volumes and speeds, particularly where distance between crossings is great, should be provided. Controls can be signals, pedestrian-actuated flashers, or other hybrid signalization.

Source: U.S. Department of Housing and Urban Development.

Table 29   Basics of a Bike-Friendly Community

- Bicyclists should have safe, convenient, and comfortable access to all destinations.

- Every street could be used by cyclists, regardless of designation or improvements.

- Not every street needs to accommodate cyclists specifically; however, parallel streets and corridor networks need to provide appropriate facilities for all abilities. Bike, pedestrian, and transit facilities should be integrated to provide a network of travel solutions.

- Bicyclists should generally be separated from pedestrians except while on multiuse paths.

- Shared use of the roadway with vehicles is acceptable along low-volume, low-speed streets.

- Conventional or buffered bike lanes should be used on medium-volume, medium-speed streets.

- High-volume, high-speed streets need to have horizontal separation (e.g., a multiuse path) or vertical separation (e.g., a roadway barrier), as commonly provided by cycle tracks. (Cycle tracks are bikeways located on or adjacent to streets where bicycle traffic is separated from motor vehicle traffic by physical barriers, such as on-street parking and landscaped islands.)

- Bikeway treatments should provide clear guidance for how a cyclist is expected to utilize the bikeway and how vehicles and cyclists should interact in a predictable manner.

- Because most bicycle trips are short, a complete network of designated bikeways should have a grid of roughly 0.5 mile (0.8 kilometer) or less.

- Attention should always be focused on intersections or segments where safety risks are high or where a segment condition changes dramatically, to the detriment of riding space.

Source: U.S. Department of Housing and Urban Development.

where people walk on average less than 1 mile (1.6 kilometers) per day (and sometimes considerably less), planners often consider walking trips of 0.5 mile (0.8 kilometer) reasonable for most errands (a distance that can be covered in about 15 minutes), with few destinations more than 1 mile (1.6 kilometer) away (a 30-minute walk). Thus, the ideal walkable neighborhood would have most destinations within a distance of 0.5–1 mile (0.8–1.6 kilometers) for most residents.

One reason that the distance people are willing to walk, on average, is not any farther is that as many as 1 in 5 Americans report having a disability, and more than half classify their disability as severe. Many of these Americans may be unable to walk more than a short distance, some may have difficulty climbing steps or maneuvering across streets and intersections, and others may require a wheelchair, cane, or walker. To help people with mobility issues, urban planners incorporate features such as level surfaces, curb ramps, and clear signage, consistent with the Americans with Disabilities Act. (Many nonprofit agencies and government offices provide assistance to residents with disabilities, such as delivering groceries and providing help getting to medical appointments.)

Sometimes cities face opposition when adding improvements like sidewalks and bicycle lanes. Here are several examples:

- Residents may be concerned that walkers and bicyclists may aggravate already-serious traffic congestion in the neighborhood, paths may invite crime if hidden from view behind trees and bushes, and some homes may lose privacy if a path is placed behind their yards.
- Fire and other emergency officials may argue that traffic-calming islands and narrow, pedestrian-friendly streets will slow emergency vehicles or cause accidents, thereby impairing their ability to respond quickly to emergency situations.
- Business owners may complain about losing parking spaces and parking lots when taken over by paths, landscaping, and street-calming elements.
- Developers may be resistant to the idea of adding sidewalks and bicycle paths that would increase their costs.

City planners have found solutions to most of these concerns by studying traffic patterns; designing streets, sidewalks, and paths carefully; and incorporating safety features, like lighting, call boxes, stoplights, and crosswalk signals. Perhaps the most important step that planners take in addressing community concerns is to get stakeholder input early in the process by scheduling public hearings and workshops. Typical stakeholders invited to these events are homeowners, business owners, school administrators, fire and police officials, families with children, older adults, people with disabilities, and bicycle advocates.

RECOMMENDATIONS FOR CITY DWELLERS

If you live in the city, take a moment to examine your neighborhood. Is there a park nearby? Are there bicycle paths and friendly streets for shopping and meeting up with friends? Are important businesses and community services located in your neighborhood, such as grocery stores, doctors' offices, schools, and libraries? Are neighborhood streets well lit and inviting, with benches and other gathering areas? If your answer is no, you are not alone. Most neighborhoods fail in most of these aspects. However, you can take steps to improve your neighborhood, perhaps by volunteering with a local community improvement organization or forming one of your own.

The best approach is to start slow with neighborhood improvements, making incremental steps that are low cost and to which few people would object. For example, work with the city to install a few bicycle racks at strategic locations, invite a bicycle-rental company to set up nearby stations, improve streetside landscaping by adding some trees or planters, and fix any uneven sidewalks. Arrange a meeting with the police to discuss safety lighting at night, and take their recommendations to the city department responsible for streetlights. (Some larger cities have their own street-lighting bureaus, and pedestrian safety is usually a high priority.) Once a few improvements have been made and people can see that you are serious about creating a walkable and bike-friendly neighborhood, begin recruiting local businesses to support your cause by donating funds or making their storefronts more inviting (e.g., adding outdoor seating for restaurants). With these improvements underway, make a strong pitch to the mayor and local politicians that their help is needed to improve roadways, sidewalks, and bicycle lanes, and be sure to emphasize studies showing that their efforts would bring economic development to the city. Most important, resist the inevitable argument that cars should take priority in urban planning, because many studies show the opposite—that healthy communities as well as strong economic development depend on walkable, bike-friendly neighborhoods.

CITY SPOTLIGHT: COPENHAGEN—THE CITY WHERE BICYCLES RULE

In this thriving metropolis, bicycle lanes connect all parts of the city, making for an easy ride to just about anywhere you want to go. But with bicycle traffic jams at some intersections and riders bumping into each other in congested lanes, the city's initiatives to encourage bicycle riding are almost too successful.

Bicycling in Copenhagen recently achieved a remarkable milestone—there are now more bicycles on the city streets than cars. About 60 percent of residents use their bikes for daily trips around town, including over 40 percent who commute to work by bicycle. (Even a majority of elected officials in the Danish parliament ride bicycles to work.) This impressive accomplishment is made possible by an extensive bike-friendly infrastructure that includes 233 miles (375 kilometers) of bikeways and a city commitment to achieve 50 percent of commutes by bicycle by 2025. Public health in the city is benefiting immensely from the physical exercise of bicycling, and by relieving many residents from the headaches caused by automobile traffic jams, mental health is benefiting, too.

Bicycles are everywhere in Copenhagen, and just about everyone rides one daily for errands, going to school, or commuting to and from work, even traveling long distances from the suburbs. Surveys of bicycle riders indicate they want to protect the environment, but their main motivation is that bicycle riding is simply the quickest and easiest way to get around town. With more bicycles than people, bicycle lanes sometimes become congested, causing delays at intersections and worries about bumping into other riders. And there are also complaints about bicycles not being allocated enough space on city roadways—during peak commuting hours, bicyclist represent over half of the in-town traffic but are allocated only one-third of the road space. The city is working to resolve these complaints, considering these types of issues to be indicative of the population's fierce commitment to bicycle riding, which is a good thing.

To facilitate bicycling in the city, a network of dedicated bicycle lanes was established so that people can travel from across the city without leaving the lanes, in most cases arriving at their destinations faster than by car or bus. Also, traffic lights are coordinated so that bicyclists riding at speeds of about 12 miles per hour (20 kilometers per hour) encounter green traffic lights all along the way, and during the winter, bicycle lanes are cleared of snow before automobile roads (an irritation to some drivers). Bicycle lanes are often planted with trees or pass through parks, making the ride more pleasant, and "cycle-superhighways" from neighboring municipalities have been developed.

Copenhagen's bicycling tradition dates back over a century, when residents discovered that bicycles were a convenient and inexpensive mode of transportation. However, in the 1960s, automobiles began taking over the streets as car ownership became more affordable for average citizens. Eventually, gridlock ensued on major thoroughfares, green areas turned into parking lots, air pollution levels escalated, and traffic accidents multiplied. Facing these challenges, visionary government leaders began building a bicycling infrastructure consisting of dedicated bike lanes, paths, and bridges over roadways and canals. As bicycling around the city became easier, people were willing to give up their cars and get a bike, and today, less than 30 percent of residents own a car.

Eventually, bicycle riding became ingrained in the city's lifestyle, as people identified bikes with freedom of movement, healthy living, and environmental sustainability. Residents were also motivated by the low cost of owning a bicycle, and the city quickly recognized that bicycle paths were much cheaper to build than major roadways for automobiles. Public perception of the positive aspects of bicycles was aided by a city-sponsored branding campaign associating bicycle riding with personal strength, health, and independence.

Emulating Copenhagen's success, London, Amsterdam, and other European cities have been implementing similar bicycling programs, as are some large metropolitan areas in other parts of the world. For example, in Mexico City, where traffic is nearly at a standstill during busy times of the day, city officials are actively promoting bicycle riding, which is helping commuters negotiate clogged intersections and congested streets over twice as fast as cars. On the other hand, some cities, like Beijing, are headed in the opposite direction. Although Beijing has a strong bicycling tradition, its rapidly growing population has recently discovered the pleasures of car ownership, viewing bicycles as symbolic of the poverty and backwardness of the past. As a result, bicycle use in China's capital city has fallen dramatically since the 1980s.

People love to ride bicycles, not only in Copenhagen, but throughout the world. What makes Copenhagen different from many other cities is its political leadership, which has made an unwavering commitment over the years to provide the infrastructure necessary to make bicycle riding a safe and efficient way to get to work or school. Not only has public health and the environment benefited, but also commercial businesses have flourished, as people have more flexibility to visit multiple stores without searching for parking spaces. Based on Copenhagen's experience creating a bicycle culture, the lesson for other cities is that if they invest in bicycling infrastructure, people will gladly give up their cars, the cities will save money through reduced roadway construction and maintenance, and commercial centers accessible by bicycle will thrive.

Water and Sanitation

Every city of any size requires a safe and accessible water supply for its residents. This requirement is so essential that most cities are located where potable water is—near rivers, lakes, or groundwater supplies. Water covers most of the earth's surface—about 70 percent—but surprising little of it is fresh. Only about 2.5 percent of the global water inventory is freshwater, and much of this is locked up in glaciers. The remainder is saltwater mostly found in the oceans, and while desalination technology can turn saltwater into freshwater by removing the salt, the process is expensive. Most desalination takes place in countries where freshwater is in short supply—the Middle East (mainly Saudi Arabia, Kuwait, the United Arab Emirates, Qatar, and Bahrain) and North Africa (mainly Libya and Algeria). The distribution of the world's freshwater supply is summarized here:

- **Icecaps and glaciers** (including permanent snow)—68.7%
- **Groundwater** (excluding saline groundwater)—30.1%
- **Surface water** (freshwater lakes, rivers, swamps)—0.3%
- **Other** (soil moisture, ground ice, permafrost, atmospheric, biological)—0.9%

Along with potable water, cities also require effective sanitation systems. "Sanitation" generally refers to the collection, treatment, and disposal (or reuse) of wastewater and human excreta, and it can also include efforts within a city to maintain hygienic conditions, such as garbage collection. Well-designed and functional sanitation systems are essential to prevent the spread of diseases, including cholera, diarrhea, dysentery, hepatitis A, typhoid, and polio, and poor sanitation is a major factor in some neglected tropical diseases, such as intestinal worms, schistosomiasis, and trachoma. The World Health Organization (WHO) estimates that 2.3 billion people today do not have basic sanitation facilities, such as toilets or latrines, and of this population, close to 900 million are believed to defecate in the open—in street gutters, behind bushes, or into open bodies of water. Furthermore, at least 10 percent of the world's population is thought to consume food that has been irrigated by unclean wastewater, potentially tainting the food supply. Among the diseases associated with poor sanitation, diarrhea alone accounts for about 300,000 deaths annually, mainly among children in developing nations.

There is a particular need for improved water and sanitation services within healthcare facilities. A recent WHO survey of healthcare facilities in 54 low- and middle-income countries is sobering, finding that 38 percent of these facilities lacked access to even rudimentary levels of water and 19 percent lacked basic sanitation. Additionally, 35 percent did not even have water and soap for handwashing. An estimated 15 percent of patients in these countries develop one or more infections during a hospital stay, including sepsis and other serious infections among newborns, causing over 400,000 deaths annually. These conditions discourage many people from seeking healthcare, including pregnant women who choose to give birth in unsanitary conditions at home. Without basic water and sanitation services in healthcare facilities that are designed to treat people who are sick, it is no wonder that infectious diseases and other illnesses are endemic in many developing countries.

The situation in developed countries is dramatically different. Most developed nations have adequate water and sanitation systems, and the spread of infectious diseases is seldom a problem. The United States has one of the world's safest water supplies, as well as sanitation systems that are among the best anywhere. Even so, contamination can occur from time to time from accidental sewage releases, naturally occurring contaminants (e.g., arsenic, uranium, and radon), and local agricultural practices that allow fertilizers, pesticides, or feedlot waste to enter the water supply. Additionally, manufacturing operations can release toxic chemicals that make their way into groundwater and surface water. Another problem concerns contaminants like lead that may leach from drinking-water pipes, as recently happened in Flint, Michigan, exposing residents to unacceptably high lead concentrations in their drinking water.

Although the United States has much to be proud of when it comes to providing a safe water supply and good sanitation for its residents, the nation has failed to ensure that adequate drinking water and sanitation are available to its American Indian and Alaska Native people. Water is sacred to many tribal nations and vital to health, cultural practices, and agriculture. Yet, legal rights to water have long been contested with surrounding states and localities, and water allocations to tribal lands are often insufficient. According to the U.S. Indian Health Service, adequate sanitation facilities are lacking in about 36 percent of American Indian and Alaska Native homes, and 6.5 percent of these homes do not have access to safe drinking water or waste disposal facilities, or both, compared with less than 1 percent of the general population.

American Indian and Alaska Native peoples have long suffered from worse health compared with other Americans, including lower life expectancy and disproportionate disease burden. This is due to a variety of causes, among them pervasive poverty, discrimination in the delivery of health services, and economic adversity. To address these disparities, the Indian Health Service has been designated the principal federal healthcare provider and health advocate for American Indian and Alaska Native people, with the goal of raising their health status to the highest possible level by ensuring that comprehensive, culturally acceptable personal and public health services are available and accessible to all.

Two events stand out in the history of municipal water and sanitation. One involved the British physician John Snow (1813–1858), who investigated cholera outbreaks in London in the mid-1800s. At the time, cholera was believed to be caused by some unknown airborne agent that spread from household to household as residents breathed the unhealthy city air. Snow was skeptical about this theory and began studying the outbreaks by carefully plotting cases of cholera on a map. Using this approach, he discovered that a serious outbreak in 1854 in the Soho district of London occurred in the vicinity of a water pump used by the cholera victims. Suspecting that contaminated water from the pump was spreading the disease, Snow asked city officials to close down the pump, which they reluctantly agreed to do as an experiment. Cholera cases began to diminish almost immediately, proving Snow's theory. (It was later discovered that a woman whose baby was sick from cholera had been washing diapers in water that she dumped into a cesspool close to the pump, resulting in the pump water becoming contaminated with cholera bacteria.) Public health historians consider that Snow's mapping technique, innovative at the time, marked the beginning of the field of epidemiology.

Another pivotal event in urban water and sanitation history occurred in 1908, when John Leal (1858–1914), a physician and a sanitary advisor to the Jersey City Water Supply Company, began adding small amounts of chlorine to the water supply in Jersey City, New Jersey. Sanitary engineers at the time were aware that certain chemicals could act as disinfectants when added to water, but there was strong resistance against adding chemicals to water-supply systems, for fear of contaminating the drinking water for potentially tens of thousands of city residents. Despite these concerns, Leal went about constructing a chlorination system, with the assistance of George Warren Fuller (1868–1934), a highly respected sanitary engineer. The experiment was remarkably successful, as demonstrated by a dramatic reduction in the city's death rate from typhoid fever and other bacterial infections, and by 1914, over half the U.S. population served by public water-supply systems was drinking chlorinated water. During the first half of the twentieth century, life expectancy in developed countries increased by 20 years, due to large part to the disinfection of drinking water and associated declines in diarrhea and other viral and bacterial diseases.

IMPACT ON URBAN HEALTH

Water and sanitation are essential to life. City residents expect their drinking water to be healthy and free from contamination, and city managers know that if the huge volumes of human waste and garbage created in urban areas are not handled properly through sewage and waste disposal systems, a public health crisis can quickly develop. The lack of clean water and proper sanitation can lead to a wide range of diseases, including diarrhea, lymphatic filariasis, Japanese encephalitis, schistosomiasis, trachoma, West Nile virus, and neglected tropical diseases such as helminth infections, caused by parasitic worms transmitted by eggs in human feces that contaminate the soil in areas where sanitation is poor. (The WHO reports that about 1.5 billion people have helminth infections worldwide.) Water contaminants can also lead to various gastrointestinal illnesses, reproductive problems, and neurological disorders. As is often the case with threats to human health, the populations at greatest risk from poor water quality and inadequate sanitary conditions are young children, pregnant women, older adults, and people with compromised immune systems.

Unsanitary conditions, particularly in developing countries, have been linked to "stunting," which is the impaired growth and development experienced by children due to repeated infections, as well as poor nutrition and insufficient psychosocial stimulation. (The WHO considers children stunted if their height is more than two standard deviations below the median for their age.) Stunting is associated with poor cognition and school performance, low adult wages and productivity, and increased risk of nutrition-related diseases later in life. Common mechanisms for stunting include repeated cases of diarrhea, helminth infections, and environmental enteric dysfunction, a syndrome of inflammation and reduced absorptive capacity and barrier function in the small intestine. (Environmental enteric dysfunction is associated with poor sanitation, as well as certain intestinal infections and micronutrient deficiencies, and it is widespread in low- and middle-income countries.)

The absence of safe sanitation systems in some cities in developing countries has been linked with another troubling phenomenon—antimicrobial resistance. This occurs when medicines, such as antibiotics, antifungals, antivirals, antimalarials, and anthelmintics, are misused or overused, causing bacteria, fungi, viruses, and parasites to undergo changes (usually genetic) that allow them to become resistant to the medicines. Antimicrobial resistance limits the ability of doctors to treat common infectious diseases, and it can introduce a high risk into some medical procedures, including major surgery, diabetes management, chemotherapy, and organ transplants. The WHO reports that inadequate sanitary conditions, including unclean food-handling techniques and poor infection control, encourage the spread of antimicrobial resistance. One example of antimicrobial resistance, now occurring along the Cambodia-Thailand border region, is the resistance of *Plasmodium falciparum* (a parasite that causes a form of malaria found worldwide in tropical and subtropical areas) to almost all available antimalarial medicines. Global health professionals are very concerned that this multidrug resistance will emerge in other parts of the region as well.

The relationship between water quality, sanitation, and public health is clear, and there is no doubt that contaminated water and poor sanitation can lead to the spread of infectious diseases. Nevertheless, the data needed to quantify these relationships are not extensive and sometimes anecdotal due to difficulties in conducting randomized controlled trials (studies involving randomly selected experimental and control groups) and blind environmental interventions (where the experimenters and participants do not know who is receiving the intervention). Many studies show clear connections between water quality, sanitation, and health, and others show weaker associations, perhaps due to inconsistencies in experimental design or difficulties in intervention delivery. For these reasons, the WHO and many other health agencies continue to conduct field studies and laboratory research to understand how best to protect public health when water quality and sanitation are compromised.

WHAT CITIES ARE DOING ABOUT WATER AND SANITATION

Most cities in developed countries have well-operating water and sanitation systems that deliver clean drinking water to city residents and prevent the spread of most diseases through solid waste management and other sanitation systems. Nevertheless, these systems are not perfect, and improvements are constantly progress to replace outdated pipes and other equipment and upgrade facilities to incorporate the latest technologies and innovations. A number of municipal facilities participate in water-recycling programs, which involve reusing wastewater for beneficial purposes. Recycled wastewater is most commonly used for nonpotable purposes, which can include agricultural uses, as well as irrigation for public park landscaping and golf-course greens. Recycled wastewater is also sometimes used for cooling water at power plants and oil refineries, industrial process water, toilet flushing, dust control, and concrete mixing. There have been a number of cases where recycled wastewater meeting high water-quality standards is used for potable purposes, such as recharging groundwater aquifers and increasing the water in reservoirs. For many years, Orange County, California, has injected highly treated recycled wastewater into aquifers to prevent saltwater intrusion while adding to the potable groundwater supply.

The situation is entirely different in developing countries, where many cities and emerging towns dump untreated wastewater and human waste directly into local waterways, onto marginal lands, or into open drains in neighborhoods. Also, as these cities grow, water resources become increasingly polluted, and groundwater, when available, is sometimes depleted faster than it is replenished. The Organisation for Economic Cooperation and Development (OECD) estimates that by the middle of this century, over 40 percent of the world's population could be living in areas under severe water stress, a situation only made worse by drought and other effects of climate change.

With help from many international aid organizations, much progress has been made in improving water and sanitation systems in the developing world, but this work in increasingly undermined by rapid urban population growth and increasing pollution. Many large cities do not have treatment plants, or the plants are undersized and unable to handle the growing volume of wastewater, and many urban dwellers continue practicing open defecation. On the other hand, where water and sanitation systems have been improved and updated, advances have been seen in food security, health, and economic development. Some of the water and sanitation system improvements and updates include upgrading waste collection and management strategies to minimize wastes that collect on streets and in open sewers, adding emission controls to waste incinerators or replacing the incinerators with waste recycling and reuse programs, capturing methane from treatment plants and landfills for reuse in generating heat and power, and using simple animal and sewage waste digesters to generate biogas cooking fuel.

RECOMMENDATIONS FOR CITY DWELLERS

If you live in a city in the United States or some other developed nation, you most likely have access to a clean drinking-water supply and basic sanitation services, including trash pickup and disposal. Waterborne and sanitation-related diseases occasionally occur in these urban areas, but a much more probable cause of disease is poor hygiene at home or work or exposure to bacteria and viruses in the community. These risks can be reduced with good hygiene practices, especially frequent handwashing, face washing, and bathing with soap and water. Recent research has found that many germs exist in public areas on handrails and countertops, and even on cell-phone screens. Thus, when out in public, it is always a good practice to wash your hands frequently and avoid touching your face, mouth, eyes, nose, or open sores and cuts. If soap and water are not available, the Centers for Disease Control and Prevention (CDC) recommends using hand sanitizers containing at least 60 percent alcohol, and then washing again with soap and water as soon as possible. More advice on handwashing and when to use hand sanitizers can be found in this CDC fact sheet: *Handwashing and Hand Sanitizer Use at Home, at Play, and Out and About* (https://www.cdc.gov/handwashing/pdf/hand-sanitizer-factsheet.pdf).

Clean drinking water and good hygiene are even more important in low- and middle-income countries, where it is estimated that a large percentage of foodborne disease outbreaks are spread by contaminated hands, and where good handwashing with soap and water can reduced diarrheal disease–associated deaths by up to 50 percent. Washing the hands, face, and body is also one of the most important ways to reduce the risk of infection and illness, as is access to clean drinking water. In many parts of the world, where good personal hygiene is difficult due to limited clean water and soap, alcohol-based hand sanitizers can be effective. Frequent teeth-cleaning using safe water is also important.

Research studies have established a link between poor sanitation and hygiene and serious diseases in developing countries. For example, trachoma, an eye infection responsible for the blindness or visual impairment of about 1.9 million people worldwide, can be prevented through improved facial cleanliness, using soap and water and better sanitation to reduce fly-breeding sites. Similarly, people with lymphatic filariasis, a parasitic disease caused by microscopic worms and a leading cause of permanent disability throughout the world, can prevent secondary infections and decrease the risk of elephantiasis (impaired immune function and swelling, for example, of the arms and legs) by daily washing of swollen areas with soap and water, as well as disinfecting wounds with antibacterial or antifungal cream.

Regardless of where you live, you should always practice good hygiene, including thorough handwashing and face washing, especially under the following circumstances:

• Before, during, and after preparing food, treating a cut or wound, and caring for someone who is sick
• Before eating food, especially when using your hands
• After using the toilet, blowing your nose, coughing, sneezing, contacting garbage, touching an animal or animal waste, and changing diapers or cleaning up a child who has used the toilet

Extra care is required for workers who routinely handle "biosolids," the organic residues resulting from the treatment of commercial, industrial, and municipal wastewater (i.e., sewage). Contact with biosolids may occur at the sewage treatment plant or during application of biosolids as soil conditioners. Precautions include thorough handwashing, eating in designated areas away from biosolid-handling activities, wearing clothing that prevents contact with biosolids (e.g., coveralls, boots, gloves, goggles, respirators, and face shields), removing biosolids from footwear before entering a vehicle or building, changing into clean clothing at the end of the workday, and using gloves to prevent skin abrasion. Workers should also consult their physicians about the need for vaccinations (e.g., against tetanus, polio, typhoid fever, and hepatitis A and B).

Workplace Health and Safety

Unless you are independently wealthy, you will probably spend most of your adult life working. Even if you are in school, you may have a part-time job, and older adults are remaining in the workforce longer than any time in the past, often well into their 70s and 80s. Some people work from home, but most workers perform their jobs elsewhere, perhaps in an office building, store, restaurant, or factory. No matter where you work, you risk being exposed to agents or situations than can threaten your health and safety. In the city, these concerns are usually greater at industrial facilities and manufacturing plants, where hazardous materials may be handled and machinery can cause injury. However, unhealthy or unsafe working conditions can also be found at commercial operations, warehouses, and even office buildings, and outdoor construction and highway workers are also at risk.

Understanding occupational health and safety is important because people spend so much of their time at work—often 8–10 hours a day, or about a third of their workday life. And while workers are usually considered among the healthiest segments of society, they are also exposed to more hazards, leading to injury and disease. Among the world's 3 billion workers, 85 percent live in less-developed countries, where work protections are often minimal or nonexistent. Whereas 50 percent or more of the workers in many developed countries have access to adequate occupational health and safety protections and services, this figure may be as low as 5–10 percent in developing countries.

The International Labour Organization (a United Nations agency representing 187 member-states) reports that almost 3 million people die every year from occupational accidents and work-related diseases, and over 350 million nonfatal work-related injuries and illnesses occur annually. Many of these injuries and illnesses result in extended absences from work, and if the injured employees lack workers' compensation, disability, or health insurance benefits, a serious injury or illness can have devastating economic consequences for the workers and their families, including loss of job. Employers also suffer from loss of skilled workers, early retirements, absenteeism, and insurance premium increases when their workers are injured or get sick on the job. It is estimated that the economic burden of poor occupational health and safety practices approaches 4 percent of the annual global gross domestic product.

In the United States, about 3 million workplace injuries and illnesses and 5,000 fatal work injuries are reported annually. Injuries and illnesses are commonly associated with transportation incidents (the most common cause of fatalities); violence and other injuries by people or animals (including workplace homicides and suicides); injuries from slips, trips, and falls; contact with dangerous objects and equipment; exposure to harmful substances or environments; fires and explosions; and alcohol use and overdoses from nonmedical use of drugs while on the job. U.S. occupations with significant fatality rates include truck driving, the construction trades, road maintenance and repair, farming and other agricultural work, landscaping and grounds maintenance, refuse collecting, roof installing, heavy industry manufacturing (e.g., iron and steel production), logging, and protective-service occupations, including police officers. About 20 percent of work-related fatalities in the United States are among foreign-born workers, often from Mexico, and nearly 95 percent of fatalities are among males.

Injury and death from workplace violence have become a growing problem, with well over 1 million incidents every year in the United States. Most workplace violence is associated with criminal intent, such as robbery and shoplifting, but violence also occurs between workers and customers, clients, patients, students, and inmates. Disgruntled workers with a score to settle and domestic violence that spills over into the workplace are other causes. The risk of workplace violence is higher for workers who interact with the public, handle money or valuables, work alone, and work late at night, and the highest risk for nonfatal assaults occurs in nursing homes, social services offices, hospitals, grocery stores, restaurants, and bars. High-risk professions for homicide include taxi drivers, liquor- and jewelry-store workers, detectives and protective-service personnel (including police), and gas-station attendants.

Since the beginning of the Industrial Revolution, worker injuries have been frequent, initially occurring at mining operations and later at iron and steel plants, cotton mills, and textile factories. Later, especially in the twentieth century, health professionals began to understand the seriousness of job-related illnesses and diseases caused by exposure to heavy metals like mercury and lead, coal and silica dust, asbestos, toxic chemicals, radioactive substances, and infectious agents. In the United States, to address these concerns in a comprehensive manner, the Occupational Safety and Health Act of 1970 was enacted to ensure that employers provide a workplace free from hazards to health and safety, such as exposure to toxic chemicals, excessive noise levels, mechanical dangers, heat and cold stress, and unsanitary conditions. The Act also created the Occupational Safety and Health Administration (OSHA) and National Institute for Occupational Safety and Health. Most developed nations also have rigorous worker protection laws, and the workers' health program and global plan of action by the World Health Organization (WHO) address all aspects of worker health.

In the early twentieth century, no one person did more to raise concerns about worker health and safety than Alice Hamilton, who is often considered the founding mother of the field of occupational medicine. Back then, employees in factories and mines worked long hours and were routinely exposed to dangerous fumes and serious safety hazards. Hamilton sneaked into American factories and mines without permission to study and document working conditions, exposing the dangers in pottery and printing plants, smelting operations, steel plants, mines, and munitions factories. Additionally, she researched the health risks associated with occupational exposure to many toxic substances, including lead, carbon monoxide, phosphorus, benzene, and picric acid. Through this work, she is credited with preventing countless deaths from lead poisoning, cancer, black lung disease, anemia, and factory accidents. In 1919, upon becoming the first female faculty member at Harvard Medical School (a quarter-century before female students would be admitted) and facing unsympathetic critiques from the news media, she remarked, "Yes, I am the first woman on the Harvard faculty—but not the first one who *should* have been appointed."

IMPACT ON URBAN HEALTH

About 95 percent of occupational health and safety complaints are associated with on-the-job injuries, which are usually minor in nature, such as cuts, scratches, and bruises. However, injuries occasionally are much more serious, like the loss of an eye or limb or a traumatic head injury. Sprains, strains, and tears account for the largest number of injuries where a worker has to miss a day or more at work, and within this category, the most common site of injury is the back. It is no surprise that back pain is frequently reported among workers who lift heavy objects, but it is also unusually common with office workers, many of whom may not have access to ergonomically designed chairs and other furniture. Teenagers working part-time jobs after school are also susceptible to injuries, especially when they are involved with agriculture, construction, landscaping, grounds-keeping, or lawn service, or if they operate equipment like forklifts and tractors.

While the vast majority of occupational health and safety issues involve minor injuries, occupational illnesses can sometimes be very serious and even life-threatening. There are four common types of occupational illnesses. Most frequently reported are musculoskeletal disorders, which include injuries to muscles, tendons, ligaments, nerves, joints, bones, and the supporting vascular system. The most common musculoskeletal disorder is repeated trauma disorder, a familiar example being carpal tunnel syndrome, a compression of the median nerve in the wrist and hand often attributed to repetitive motions like typing. (It may also be caused by external injuries to the wrist and hand and other health conditions.) Symptoms of carpal tunnel syndrome include pain, numbness, tingling, weak grip, occasional clumsiness, and a tendency to drop things.

A second type of occupational illness involves skin diseases and disorders, which include dermatitis (inflammation usually involving an itchy rash on skin that is swollen and reddened), eczema (a chronic form of dermatitis that may flare up periodically and cause dry and scaly skin, itching, red or brownish-gray patches, and small, raised bumps), and chemical burns (also known as "caustic burns," which may occur from exposure to irritants, such as chemical acids and bases). Skin diseases and disorders are more frequent in the agriculture, forestry, and fishing industries, but these health issues can also occur in other manufacturing and commercial operations where chemicals may come in contact with the skin.

A third occupational illness category is noise-induced hearing loss and tinnitus (ringing in the ears), often caused by repeated exposure to loud sounds in manufacturing plants or at construction sites. Hearing loss can limit the ability to understand speech and communicate, and loud noises at work can cause psychological stress, limit concentration, decrease productivity, and contribute to workplace accidents. OSHA reports that 22 million American workers are exposed to potentially damaging noise at work each year, and nearly $250 million is spent annually on worker compensation for hearing-loss disability.

The final category of occupational illness is respiratory disorder, which includes a range of hazards due to the inhalation of toxic substances, such as work-related asthma, chronic bronchitis and emphysema, chronic obstructive pulmonary disease, pneumoconiosis, black lung disease, asbestosis, silicosis, and byssinosis. Sometimes cancer and reproductive disorders can also occur, and occasionally respiratory disease results in severe disability or death.

In addition to these four common categories of occupational disease, other diseases may result from exposure to poisons and pesticides, infectious agents, toxic gases, pharmaceuticals, and nanomaterials encountered in the workplace. These health hazards may be made worse with repeated exposures or with concomitant exposures to other agents.

A group of people whose health and safety concerns are often neglected are migrant workers, who are often employed in hazardous jobs, working under worse conditions and for less pay than other workers. Furthermore, migrants frequently have limited access to healthcare and experience language or cultural barriers, and they may be subjected to human rights violations, abuse, human trafficking, and violence. Globally, around 250 million people are believed to be transnational migrants (traveling between countries), and about half of this population is working, often in construction or hospitality jobs in the city or as farm workers. Migrant workers frequently suffer from adverse occupational exposures, injuries, and even fatalities, and many are reluctant to seek help because of their documentation status or fear of retaliation.

WHAT CITIES ARE DOING ABOUT WORKPLACE HEALTH AND SAFETY

Most cities do not have strong worker health and safety laws, in part because health and safety regulations are often implemented at the federal and state levels of government. For example, in the United States, the Occupational Safety and Health Act mandates strong worker protections that apply to most private and public employers and workers nationwide. The general duty clause of the Act requires employers to comply with health and safety standards and to furnish each employee with a workplace "free from recognized hazards that are causing or are likely to cause death or serious physical harm." Many other developed nations also have similar general-duty requirements, but the same cannot be said for developing nations, where worker protections are limited or entirely absent at both the national and state levels and within individual cities.

Although companies and workers in many cities fall under the umbrella of national and state health and safety regulations, some cities supplement these regulations with their own requirements. For example, local construction permits may require builders to demonstrate compliance with federal and state occupational safety laws, and evidence of worker compensation and disability insurance may also be required. Also, builders may be required to provide safety training to their workers, meet fire and ventilation codes, and follow safety rules for asbestos and lead paint removal and disposal when renovating or demolishing buildings. Also, city officials may perform safety inspections at certain facilities, such as swimming pools and day-care facilities, and regulations may be enacted on specific types of businesses, like nail salons. Some cities are required by state law to have in place a workplace accident and injury reduction program, and larger cities ordinarily hire one or more health and safety professionals, such as those listed in Table 30, to implement city health and safety programs and ensure compliance with applicable policies and regulations.

Cities are also responsible for ensuring that their own employees (i.e., workers on the city payroll) work under safe conditions, and that city offices and other public facilities are in compliance with applicable occupational health and safety regulations. Examples of public facilities subject to health and safety regulations are water and wastewater treatment plants, trash and recycling operations, health clinics, public housing developments, police and fire departments, libraries, schools, and public swimming pools. Cities are also responsible for protecting employees who work outdoors, such as landscaping and road maintenance workers. Larger cities sometimes provide training to employees on conflict resolution, drug and alcohol abuse, motor vehicle safety, and steps to prevent back injuries, and emergency response personnel may be trained in how to respond to and protect themselves from leaks and spills of hazardous materials in emergencies.

Table 30   Occupational Health and Safety Professionals

Profession	Responsibilities
Health physicist	Monitors radiation in the workplace and develops plans to respond to accidental releases of radioactive materials and potential exposures to workers.
Industrial hygienist	Evaluates environmental factors, such as fumes, excessive noise, poor lighting, and insufficient ventilation, which can lead to illness; and establishes controls to prevent exposure or reduce it to safe levels.
Occupational health nurse	Focuses on health education and illness prevention, as well as providing first aid and running the company clinic, if any.
Occupational physician	Specializes in worker health and safety and evaluates and treats occupational illnesses and injuries. (Except in the largest companies, this person is likely to be a consultant rather than an employee and located off site at a medical center.)
Safety professional	Detects and protects against physical hazards in the workplace that can cause injury.

Source: J. F. McKenzie and R. R. Pringer, *An Introduction to Community and Public Health* (Burlington, MA: Jones and Bartlett Learning, 2015).

To reduce the risk of injuries to employees, the following actions are often considered standard practice for both public- and private-sector employers:

- Conducting a hazard inventory to identify any physical, chemical, biological, or psychological hazards in the workplace
- Studying the likelihood of future adverse events, like leaks or explosions, and implementing measures to prevent such events
- Installing engineering controls, such as new equipment, barriers, and modified processes, to minimize or eliminate hazards

- Implementing a monitoring and surveillance program to detect hazards before they become serious
- Ensuring that employees take safety training and have personal safety equipment appropriate to their jobs, and providing a medical-monitoring program to those employees with the potential for exposure to hazardous substances

Similarly, to reduce the risk of an employee developing an occupational disease, the following actions are commonly followed in both government offices and private companies:

- Establishing good employee hygiene habits, including rigorous handwashing, and insisting that employees stay home when not feeling well
- Determining if less toxic substitutes are available for any hazardous substances used in the workplace
- Ensuring that employees are well trained and have the proper personal protective devices (e.g., protective work suits, gloves, safety shoes, and respirators) to avoid exposure to hazardous materials and other toxic agents
- Installing ventilation hoods, air-cleaning systems, and other engineering controls to prevent inhalation exposure to disease-causing agents
- Testing regularly for exposure to toxic gases and particulates, radon, and any radioactive sources
- Performing routine medical screenings (particularly for employees handling dangerous materials), conducting regular health education and promotion events, and investing in employee health (via such offerings as free gym memberships and smoking cessation programs).
- Scheduling independent, third-party audits to ensure that the facility is in compliance with all health and safety regulations, and following standard protocols for preventing exposure to toxic, disease-causing agents.

Table 31 (chemical exposure in a nail salon), Table 32 (noise exposure in a factory), and Table 33 (injuries among restaurant workers) present case studies illustrating several common workplace hazards in the city, as well as steps to protect worker health and safety.

RECOMMENDATIONS FOR CITY DWELLERS

People who work in the city may be exposed to occupational hazards that they may not even be aware of, such as toxic gases that they cannot see or smell, a slick spot on the floor, or a virus lurking around the break room. Even if they work in an office building, hazards may be present, such as off-gassing of volatile organic compounds from paint and furniture, poor lighting, or unstable office furniture. Some effects may be obvious, but others, like hearing loss, may build up over time and may not be apparent for a number of years. For people who both work and live in the city, their occupational hazards may be compounded by air or water pollution or loud noises they encounter around town—a jackhammer used on road repair work, a subway train screeching to a stop, or a boom box playing some-one's loud music. Here are some tips that urban dwellers can follow to protect their health and safety:

- Be alert and aware at work and in public places, and watch for obvious concerns like slick spots and tripping hazards.

- If there is a health-and-safety program at work, learn about any work-place hazards, ways to protect yourself, and any health-monitoring programs. In particular, do not be shy about wearing recommended personal protection equipment, such as protective clothing, safety shoes, ear protection, and respirators.

- Even if your company offers a health-and-safety program, routinely check your surroundings and do not take anything for granted. (For example, if you have to shout to be heard by a coworker or hear ringing or humming in your ears when leaving work, your workplace may have a noise problem.)

- Have regular checkups with your doctor, including baseline blood tests, and consider getting all recommended vaccinations.

- Carry ear protection with you (e.g., earplugs or earmuffs) if you expect to be in a noisy environment, including a loud concert.

Of course, you should strive to live a healthy lifestyle—void of drugs, alcohol abuse, and tobacco—because a healthy body is better prepared to protect itself against workplace illnesses and injuries. As the slogan goes, "Workplace safety does not happen by accident—it begins with you!"

Table 31   Case Study—Chemical Exposure in a Nail Salon

Hazard	Products used in nail salons contain chemicals that could affect the health of workers, particularly when exposed repeatedly over days, weeks, or months of employment.
Routes of exposure	Exposure could occur by inhalation of vapors or dust, skin or eye contact with chemicals, or ingestion through contaminated food or cigarettes. Exposure may be worse if ventilation is poor.
Toxic agents	Some potentially hazardous chemicals that may be used in nail salons include acetone (nail polish remover), acetonitrile (fingernail glue remover), dibutyl phthalate (nail polish), ethyl acetate (nail polish, nail polish remover, fingernail glue), ethyl methacrylate (artificial nail liquid), formaldehyde (nail polish, nail hardener), isopropyl acetate (nail polish, nail polish remover), methacrylic acid (nail primer), methyl methacrylate (artificial nail products, although banned for use in many states), quaternary ammonium compounds (disinfectants), and toluene (nail polish, fingernail glue).
Health effects	Depending on the chemical and on the level and duration of exposure, adverse health effects could include allergic reactions, asthma, breathing difficulties, concentration problems, coughing, dizziness, dry or cracked skin, exhaustion, fainting, headaches, irritation (of eyes, skin, nose, mouth, and throat), loss of smell, nausea, numbness, skin burns, sleepiness, vomiting, weakness, and wheezing. Long-term, repeated, or high-level exposure may cause other serious health concerns, including cancer, liver and kidney damage, and harm to an unborn child during pregnancy.
Actions to protect workers' health and safety	Choose safer, less toxic products when available. Determine if respirator protection is needed (usually not required if good ventilation is provided; if required, use a high-quality respirator designed for removal of gases and particles—surgical masks, even when stuffed with tissue, are ineffective).

Table 31   (continued)

	Install and operate an excellent ventilation system (the best way to lower chemical concentrations in a salon other than eliminating use of the chemicals altogether).
	Read the product-safety statement on product labels and safety data sheets.
	Require workers to report any health issues or symptoms of exposure.
	Use safe work practices to avoid regular and accidental exposures (e.g., close bottles tightly, use metal trash cans with tightly closing lids, use only the amount of product needed, closely follow instructions for use and disposal, wash hands before eating and drinking and prior to applying cosmetics, and do not eat or store food in work areas).
	Wear gloves and long-sleeved shirts and goggles to keep products away from skin and eyes.

Source: OSHA.

Table 32   Case Study—Noise Exposure in a Factory

Hazard	Loud, repeated noise can cause permanent hearing loss. It can also reduce productivity and present a safety hazard by interfering with concentration and communication. Noise-induced hearing loss is one of the most common occupational illnesses.
Sources of exposure	Sources include air jets, blasting and crushing operations, conveying systems, electric motors and engines, milling machines and grinders, pneumatic tools, pumps and compressors, transportation systems, ventilator and exhaust fans, and woodworking machines.
Actions to protect workers' health and safety	**Engineering controls**—modifying or replacing equipment or other physical changes, such as choosing low-noise tools and machinery, thoroughly lubricating equipment, installing sound barriers, and enclosing or isolating the sources of loud sounds.

Table 32   (continued)

	Administrative controls—changing workplace conditions, including operating equipment during shifts where fewer people are exposed, limiting the amount of time that workers are exposed to loud noises, requiring workers to maintain a safe distance from noisy operations, and providing quiet areas where hearing can recover.
	Hearing protection—requiring workers to wear hearing protection, such as high-quality earplugs and earmuffs.
	Medical monitoring and training—performing routine hearing tests to ensure that worker hearing levels are not deteriorating, and conducting regular training on hearing protection.
	Hearing conservation program—implementing a program that identifies workers at risk from hazardous noise levels, informing workers about the risk of loud noises in their work areas, conducting noise sampling and allowing workers to observe these tests, maintaining a worker audiometric testing program, implementing follow-up procedures for workers showing hearing loss, providing individualized hearing protection devices and training, and maintaining records of noise monitoring, hearing tests, and actions taken to protect worker hearing.

Source: OSHA.

Table 33   Case Study—Injuries Among Restaurant Workers

Hazard	Restaurants, particularly with kitchen work, present a number of hazards to employees, such as hot equipment and oil, sharp utensils, heavy lifting, and slippery floors.
Health effects	The following are the most frequent injuries: • **Muscle strains, sprains, and tears**—from slips, trips, falls, lifting, repetitive motions, reaching, and twisting. • **Cuts and lacerations**—from knives, broken glass, and food-processing equipment, such as slicers, grinders, and mixers.

Table 33   (continued)

	• **Burns and scalds**—from hot liquids (e.g., oil and grease), heating and cooking equipment, hot pots and trays, and steam.
Actions to protect workers' health and safety	Both restaurant managers and employees have responsibilities, including the following: • **Managers**—teach employees how to do their jobs safely, check for unsafe conditions daily, clean up spills quickly, install nonslip mats in dishwashing and cooking areas, keep safety guards in place on equipment (e.g., slicers, grinders, and mixers), have a first-aid kit readily available, and post emergency numbers. • **Employees**—learn to use knives safely and store them properly, keep hands away from dangerous equipment (e.g., slicers, grinders, and mixers), allow hot oil to cool before handling, carry hot items carefully (e.g., use potholders, oven mitts, or dry towels), keep the face and hands away from steam, clean up spills quickly, and wear slip-resistant shoes. Back injuries from lifting heavy items are common. Some tips to protect yourself include bending at the hips or knees, keeping your back straight and avoiding twisting while lifting, keeping your head up and the load close to your body, using "hand holds" on boxes, and getting help moving large or heavy items.

Source: New York City Department of Health and Mental Hygiene.

EXPERT COMMENTARY: WORKER HEALTH

Labor laws, as well as health and safety protections, are difficult to monitor and enforce in nonstandard work arrangements, and there are numerous stories of labor violations (e.g., wage theft) and severe traumatic injuries in these unregulated jobs.

Linda Forst, Professor and Physician

University of Illinois at Chicago School of Public Health

Dr. Forst specializes in occupational health, with a focus on low-wage workers. She conducts research related to at-risk working populations and does public health surveillance for work-related illnesses and injuries. Dr. Forst teaches in the classroom about the environment, toxicology, and disease, and she also teaches an online continuing education course called the Global Program in Occupational Health Practice. In addition, she cares for workers in an urgent-care clinical setting and prepares documentation for workers' compensation insurance.

What do you see as the greatest issues regarding worker health in urban areas, what are the major obstacles to addressing these issues, and what is your hope for the future?

The migration of workers from farms to urban settings marks the late nineteenth and the twentieth centuries. Technological advances led to the Industrial Revolution, with a growth in manufacturing and coincident expansion of transportation, warehousing, shipping, and utilities; a strong and centralized financial sector; and booming commercial and residential construction. The service sector has also grown to meet the needs of centralized and expanding populations in urban environments. As we get further into the twenty-first century, we are seeing expanded trade and the offshoring of manual labor jobs, the explosion of the service sector (particularly in healthcare, education, and entertainment), and further technological advances requiring a highly skilled workforce. The squeeze on low-skilled workers is being exploited by candidates for elected office, and the blame targets immigrants who, some politicians say, will take the remaining unskilled jobs from citizens. It behooves us to find and communicate the facts and make plans for the economy and employment based on the evidence.

Another current issue is the change in employment arrangements from "standard" to "precarious" work. A standard employment arrangement describes full-time work under the employer's supervision with a contract of indefinite duration, standard working hours, and social benefits such as health insurance, medical leave, workers' compensation, pensions, and unemployment insurance. Precarious work is part time, short term, temporary, contracted, and sometimes home-based, and it often comes with low wages (such that multiple jobs are needed) and no social benefits. There is a rising segment of the population that is self-employed, telecommuting, and temporarily employed. So-called "gig economy" workers hustle wages in ride sharing, home sharing, dog walking, house cleaning, childcare, eldercare, residential construction, landscaping, and freelancing of all types. Labor laws, as well as health and safety protections, are difficult to monitor and enforce in nonstandard work arrangements, and there are numerous stories of labor violations (e.g., wage theft) and severe traumatic injuries in these unregulated jobs. The "cash" or "underground" economy is the most extreme example, where employment is unregistered, taxes are not paid, and workers are not assured that they will receive promised wages. There is a current need to strengthen labor laws and penalties to address the needs of the newest urban workforce.

APPENDIX

Steps to Healthy Urban Living

Many illnesses and adverse health conditions can be avoided through a healthy lifestyle and diet and by paying attention to the surrounding environment. Some steps to healthy urban living are listed here:

Avoid all tobacco products. This includes cigarettes, cigars, pipes, and chewing tobacco. When considering the use of e-cigarettes and vaping, consult expert studies, such as the National Academies of Sciences, Engineering, and Medicine's *Consensus Study Report: Public Health Consequences of E-cigarettes* (see the "Directory of Resources").

If you consume alcohol, drink in moderation. Know your limits, and never drink and drive. Many restaurants and bars provide nonalcoholic beers and other drinks for drivers, or alternatively, you can use a share-ride or taxi service.

Stay away from illicit drugs. Also, talk with your doctor about any precautions when taking prescription painkillers and other pharmaceuticals that may lead to addiction or other side effects and do not deviate from prescribed amounts.

Eat a healthy, well-balanced diet. Include organically grown foods in your diet when possible, and avoid junk foods and sugary drinks. Study the pros and cons of pesticide-treated and genetically modified foods and make informed decisions about whether to include these in your diet.

Exercise regularly. The YMCA and local sports clubs often have indoor facilities where you can exercise at a comfortable temperature and receive advice about working out from expert trainers. Consult your doctor about the right amount of exercise for you.

Get a flu shot. To avoid getting the flu, public health professionals recommend getting a flu vaccination annually, avoiding large crowds during flu season, and washing your hands frequently. According to the Centers for Disease Control and Prevention (CDC), "while severe reactions are uncommon, you should let your doctor, nurse, clinic, or pharmacist know if you have a history of allergy or severe reaction to flu vaccine or any part of flu vaccine . . . Almost all people who get influenza vaccine have no serious problems from it."

Pay attention to the local air quality forecast. In the United States, the AirNow Air Quality Index provides forecasts as well as advice (e.g., limiting outdoor activities when air pollution exceeds a certain level). These forecasts are available online and often reported during the weather segment of local TV newscasts. For allergy sufferers, local weather reports and weather websites often carry pollen-count and other allergy information.

Practice safe food-handling techniques. To reduce the risk of food contamination, wash hands prior to handling food to avoid contamination with microorganisms and dirt, wash produce before cooking or eating to rinse off any pesticides and any other harmful contaminants, cook eggs and raw meat to the appropriate temperature to kill any microorganisms, and store food appropriately to avoid spoilage and food waste.

Be careful using household cleaners, indoor pesticides, and personal-care products. Follow the label instructions carefully, use products manufactured from nontoxic substances wherever possible, and try nonchemical methods of pest control (e.g., regular sweeping and vacuuming of food particles that can attract pests). Restrict hobby activities using glues, chemicals, and paints to well-ventilated areas.

Limit exposure to loud noises. Walk away from the noise, lower the volume, or wear ear protection, such as earplugs or earmuffs. Be careful wearing headphones and earbuds because there is increasing evidence that they can cause hearing loss if the volume is too loud.

Avoid overexposure to sunlight. Limit time spent in the midday sun, especially during the hours from 10 a.m. to 4 p.m., apply a broad-spectrum, SPF 30+ sunscreen as needed to block sun exposure, stay in the shade as much as possible, and wear wide-brimmed hats, tightly woven and loose-fitting clothing, and sunglasses that provide 100 percent protection against both UVA and UVB radiation. Be careful near water, snow, and sand, which can reflect sunlight and increase the risk of sunburn. Check the UV Index before planning outdoor activities to be sure that you are adequately protected, even on a cloudy day.

Learn about workplace hazards. If you work in the city, learn about any safety or environmental hazards at your job, including ways to protect yourself and any health-monitoring programs. Do not be shy about wearing recommended personal protection equipment, such as protective clothing, safety shoes, ear protection, and respirators.

Learn to manage stress. Develop close relationships, plan fun events to help relax and keep from taking life too seriously, avoid alcohol and drugs as remedies for your troubles, and generally, take good care of yourself—eat well, get plenty of sleep, and exercise regularly. The CDC and other national and local organizations provide excellent resources for dealing with stress, anxiety, and depression, including crisis-intervention centers and hotlines. In the United States, the National Suicide Prevention Lifeline is 800-273-TALK (800-273-8255), and you can chat online at https://suicidepreventionlifeline.org.

Be connected socially. Spend time regularly with family and friends and share with them your joys and concerns. Make new friends by joining social clubs, service organizations, or faith groups in your neighborhood. Volunteering in your community can also help develop social contacts while providing the good feeling of helping someone in need. Cultivate personal relationships with a counselor, member of the clergy, or health professional to turn to for advice when problems arise.

Be on the lookout for criminal activity. When out at night, walk with a purpose, look like you know where you are going, do not ask people on the street for directions, and avoid talking on your cell phone because it can signal criminals that you are distracted and may not see them approach you. Whenever possible, go out with a friend or a group of friends.

Some organizations recommend caution with cell-phone use. To reduce radio-frequency radiation near your body, the CDC offers these tips: (1) get a hands-free headset that connects directly to your phone; (2) use the speakerphone feature more often; and (3) if you have a pacemaker and are concerned about how your cell-phone use may affect it,

contact your healthcare provider. The CDC states that there is no scientific evidence that provides a definite answer as to whether cell-
phone use causes cancer, and more research is needed before we know
if using cell phones causes health effects. (See the "Radiation Sources"
entry to learn more about safe cell-phone use.)

Glossary

Acute illness
An illness with rapid onset, as distinguished from a chronic disease that is long lasting.

Addiction
A brain disease characterized by compulsive use of a drug, alcohol, or other substance despite harmful consequences. People with addiction have an intense focus on using the addictive substance, to the point where it takes over their lives. (*See also* Substance abuse.)

Ageism
A term coined in the late 1960s to describe the prevalent age-based stereotyping, prejudice, and discrimination against older people.

Aging society
The phenomenon where as people live longer and birth rates decline, the proportion of older adults in the population increases.

Air pollutants
Contaminants in the air that can threaten health, as well as damaging crops and materials. The U.S. Environmental Protection Agency (EPA) recognizes six common air pollutants—carbon monoxide, nitrogen dioxide, lead, ozone, particulate matter, and sulfur dioxide—that are widespread in many large urban areas and can cause both immediate and longer-term health effects. (*See also* Air toxics and Hazardous air pollutants.)

Air toxics
Air pollutants known to cause cancer or other serious health effects. Air toxics are also known as *hazardous air pollutants*. (*See also* Air pollutants and Hazardous air pollutants.)

Allergen
A substance that can cause an allergic reaction because of an individual's sensitivity to the substance.

Ambient air
Outdoor air that people breathe, which can contain air pollutants.

Americans with Disabilities Act
An act of Congress that prohibits discrimination against people with disabilities in several areas, including employment, transportation, public accommodations, communications, and access to state and local government programs and services.

Antibiotic resistance
When bacteria develop the ability to defeat the drugs designed to kill them, allowing the bacteria to multiply.

Bacteria
Complex, single-cell organisms that can reproduce on their own and are responsible for a number of common illnesses, such as strep throat, urinary tract infection, and tuberculosis.

Best practice
A professional procedure that is generally accepted as correct or most effective (e.g., equipment sterilization procedures used in health clinics or food storage procedures in the restaurant business).

Bike-friendly neighborhood
An area of a city that provides bicycle lanes, pathways, and other infrastructure allowing bicyclists to make reasonably steady progress, such as commuting to work across town, without endangering themselves or others.

Bike score
A number between 0 and 100 that measures the bicycle-friendliness of a city or any address, neighborhood, or ZIP code within the city, based on an analysis of infrastructure, hills, destinations, road connectivity, and number of bike commuters. The website walkscore.com offers information about how to find the bike score of your area.

Body mass index (BMI)
A measure of body fat for adult men and women that takes into account height and weight.

Built environment
The human-created buildings, parks, and spaces within a city where people live and work.

Carbon dioxide (CO_2)
A colorless, odorless, and nontoxic gas formed by the combustion of carbon-containing fuels, such as coal, oil, and natural gas, and the principal gas contributing to climate change.

Carcinogen
A substance known or suspected to cause cancer.

Chronic disease
A long-lasting disease, as distinguished from an acute illness having a rapid onset.

Climate change
Any significant change in the measures of climate that lasts for an extended period of time (e.g., decades or longer), such as changes in temperature, precipitation, sea level, and wind patterns. (*See also* Global warming.)

Cohousing
An intentional community usually consisting of private homes, condominiums, or apartments clustered around a shared space, which may include gardens, walkways, and a common house for communal meals, meetings, and events. (Cohousing communities share the common goal of promoting social interaction and support for their members.)

Communicable disease
A disease spread from one person to another through, for example, contacting blood and bodily fluids, inhaling an airborne virus, or being bitten by an infected insect.

Cookstove
A small combustion stove that often burns wood, coal, or dung and can lead to high air pollution levels when used indoors for cooking or room heating.

Decibel (dB)
A scale for expressing the relative intensity of sounds, where the higher the decibel level, the louder the sound.

Deforestation
The large-scale clearing of forests taking place in some parts of the world that contributes to climate change. Forests help reduce climate change by removing carbon dioxide (CO_2) from the atmosphere.

Denial
The condition experienced by drug users where they do not believe they have a problem, despite strong evidence to the contrary.

Detoxification
A process that helps rid the body of harmful substances while withdrawal symptoms are being treated.

Dioxin
A term referring to a group of chemical compounds with similar chemical and biological characteristics that bioaccumulate in the food chain, persist in the environment, and can be highly toxic. (The most toxic form is 2,3,7, 8-tetrachlorodibenzo-p-dioxin, also known as TCDD.)

Drug
A generic reference to a variety of prescription, nonprescription, and illicit substances, some of which can affect behavior and potentially become addictive. (Alcohol is a drug, along with the nicotine in tobacco products and the caffeine in beverages like coffee.)

Drug Abuse Resistance Education (DARE)
A police officer–led series of classroom lessons that teach children from kindergarten through 12th grade how to resist peer pressure and live drug- and violence-free lives.

Electromagnetic radiation
A form of energy produced by electric and magnetic fields oscillating at right angles to each other. Electromagnetic radiation takes many forms and is all around us, such as television signals, radio-frequency waves, sunlight, ultraviolet (UV) radiation, and X-rays.

Environmental justice
The field of study concerned with people disproportionately exposed to pollution that can affect their health.

Environmental refugees
People forced to flee their homeland due to changes in the environment around them (e.g., prolonged drought or sea-level rise).

Epidemic
A disease outbreak that spreads quickly and affects many individuals, but not as widespread as a pandemic. (*See also* Pandemic.)

Epidemiology
The study of the frequencies, patterns, and causes of health and disease in human populations.

Food desert
An area within a city where it is difficult to buy affordable, good-quality food.

Glare
Bright light that is distracting and can cause visual discomfort. Automobile headlights are often a source of bothersome glare.

Global warming
The recent and ongoing rise in global average temperature near the earth's surface caused by increasing concentrations of greenhouse gases (GHGs) in the atmosphere. Global warming is only one aspect of climate change. (*See also* Climate change.)

Greenhouse gas (GHG)
An atmospheric gas, such as carbon dioxide (CO_2), methane, nitrous oxide, or ozone, that contributes to climate change and often originates with electric-power generation and other human activities.

Greenway
A corridor of undeveloped land planted with shade trees and other greenery.

Hazardous air pollutants
Air pollutants known to cause cancer or other serious health impacts. Hazardous air pollutants are also known as *air toxics*. (*See also* Air pollutants and Air toxics.)

Health physicist
An environmental health professional who monitors radiation in the workplace and develops plans for accidental releases of radioactive materials and potential exposure to workers.

Heat island effect
The tendency of urban areas, because of their dense materials (e.g., asphalt, brick, concrete, steel, and stone), to heat up faster and hold their heat longer than rural areas.

Heat wave
A period of several days or longer when temperatures are well above average and high enough to cause heat-related illnesses, such as heat exhaustion, heat cramps, and heatstroke (also known as *sunstroke*).

Hedonic tone
A subjective judgment about whether an odor is pleasant or unpleasant. A variety of factors influence hedonic tone, including the odor intensity, character, duration, frequency of occurrence, location, and time of day.

Hospital-acquired infection
An infection sometimes acquired by patients of hospitals, clinics, nursing homes, and rehabilitation centers while being treated for another condition. Healthcare workers can also be affected.

Immigrant
A person who comes to a country to take up permanent residence.

Industrial hygiene
A professional field concerned with protecting the health and safety of workers while on the job.

Industrial hygienist
An environmental health professional who evaluates environmental factors, such as fumes, excessive noise, and poor lighting and ventilation, that can lead to illness, and who establishes controls to reduce or prevent exposure.

Infectious disease
A human disorder caused by bacteria, viruses, fungi, parasites, and other organisms that grow and multiply in the body. Some infectious diseases are passed from person to person, while others are transmitted by insect or animal bites or by consuming contaminated food or water. (*See also* Zoonotic disease.)

Ionizing radiation
A form of radiation, such as alpha and beta particles, gamma rays, X-rays, and neutrons, that is powerful enough to produce ions by breaking molecular bonds and displacing electrons from atoms and molecules. Ionizing radiation has many useful medical applications, but repeated or high levels of exposure of it can damage tissues, alter deoxyribonucleic acid (DNA), and cause cancer.

Kodokushi
A term used in Japan (which translates into English as "isolation death") to describe situations where socially isolated older adults are found dead by neighbors, days or weeks after the death occurred.

Leadership in Energy and Environmental Design (LEED)
An internationally recognized green-building certification system providing third-party verification that a building or community is designed and built using strategies aimed at improving sustainability with regard to metrics such as energy and water use, carbon dioxide (CO_2) emissions, indoor environmental quality, and stewardship of resources.

Legionnaires' disease
A type of pneumonia caused by the *Legionella* bacteria, which can grow and spread in showers, faucets, and mechanical devices, such as plumbing systems, water tanks and heaters, and commercial air conditioning units.

Life expectancy
A statistical measure of how long a person is expected to live, taking into account factors such as sex, nationality, and lifestyle.

Light trespass
Light that spreads into areas where it is neither needed nor wanted (e.g., a security light that shines into a neighbor's bedroom window).

Macronutrients
The fats, carbohydrates, and proteins that people need to eat in relatively large amounts. Too few macronutrients can cause malnutrition and developmental problems in children, whereas too many macronutrients can cause obesity and related diseases, such as heart disease and diabetes.

Macrostressor
A major life event that causes emotional or physical tension. Macrostressors can be negative, such as divorce or loss of a job, or positive, such as marriage or getting a new job.

Microbial
A microorganism or other biological contaminant, including viruses, fungi, mold, bacteria, pollen, dander, and mites.

Micronutrients
The vitamins and minerals that people need only in small amounts, although consuming enough micronutrients is essential because they are critical

building blocks for the proteins and hormones required for proper bodily function.

Microstressor
A relatively small stress experienced while going about one's daily routine, such as getting to work on time, preparing for an exam in school, or being stuck in traffic. The buildup of microstressors can wear you down over time and affect your self-worth and confidence.

Migrant
A person who moves around regularly to find work (e.g., harvesting crops or working in construction).

Nicotine
The addictive substance found naturally in tobacco.

Nonionizing radiation
Radiation that excites atoms (i.e., causes them to move around and vibrate), but is not strong enough to dislodge them from their atomic orbits. High levels of nonionizing radiation can increase the temperature of a substance, such as in the way that a microwave oven thaws a frozen dinner and warms leftovers.

Norovirus
A highly contagious virus that causes acute gastroenteritis (inflammation of the stomach or intestines or both), leading to diarrhea, vomiting, dehydration, nausea, stomach pain, and sometimes fever, headache, and body aches. (In the United States, about half of all food-related illnesses are caused by *Norovirus*.)

Odor threshold
The lowest concentration of a substance in the air that can be detected with the human nose. Substances have various odor thresholds, and people often have different sensitivities for detecting odors.

Opioids
Defined by the National Institute on Drug Abuse as "a class of drugs that include the illegal drug heroin, synthetic opioids such as fentanyl, and pain relievers available legally by prescription, such as oxycodone (OxyContin), hydrocodone (Vicodin), codeine, morphine, and many others."

Ozone
A molecule comprising three oxygen atoms that is formed by a chemical reaction between nitrogen oxides and volatile organic compounds in the presence of sunlight. Ground-level ozone is a harmful air pollutant,

whereas ozone in the stratosphere helps block the sun's harmful ultraviolet (UV) radiation.

Pandemic
A disease outbreak that is more widespread than an epidemic, affecting a large segment of a population over a wide geographical area. (*See also* Epidemic.)

Particulate matter (PM)
A form of air pollution consisting of a complex mixture of particles and liquid droplets of many sizes, some of which may be small enough to be inhaled into lower regions of the lungs, where lung disease can occur.

Peer counseling
Where students share problems among themselves in a safe, nonjudgmental environment, often helping each other cope with abuse and addiction problems involving themselves, their friends, or loved ones at home.

Posttraumatic stress disorder (PTSD)
A mental health condition represented by an emotional and sometimes physical response to a traumatic event that was experienced or witnessed. Symptoms may include flashbacks, nightmares, severe anxiety, and uncontrollable thoughts about the event.

Potable water
Water safe for drinking.

Radioactivity
The emission of alpha or beta particles or gamma rays from radioactive elements like uranium, polonium, and radium. (It is also known as *radioactive decay*.)

Radon
A radioactive gas that forms naturally from the decay of radioactive elements found in some soil, rock, and building materials, such as brick, gypsum, and concrete.

Refugee
A person who has been forced to flee her or his country because of persecution, war, or violence.

Relapse
The recurrence of symptoms, such as when a person in recovery from addiction cannot resist the urge to drink or use drugs again after a period of abstinence.

Risk assessment
A determination of the likelihood of an event, such as the probability of contracting a disease following exposure to an infectious agent or toxic pollutant.

Safety professional
An engineer or technician who detects and takes measures to protect against physical hazards in the workplace that can cause injury.

Sanitation
Generally refers to the collection, treatment, and disposal (or reuse) of wastewater and human excreta, and it can also include efforts within a city to maintain hygienic conditions, such as garbage collection.

Secondhand smoke
Tobacco smoke exhaled by a smoker or given off by a tobacco product and inhaled by someone nearby. (It is also called *passive smoke.*)

Sick building syndrome
A term used to describe the headache, nausea, fatigue, and other ill health that occupants sometimes experience while inside a building.

Sky glow
A brightening of the sky over urban areas due to the collective contribution of light from thousands of streetlights and other sources.

Slums
Areas characterized by the World Health Organization (WHO) as "vast islands of informal economies, social exclusion, poor housing, and underdevelopment."

Smog
A mixture of ground-level pollutants, primarily consisting of ozone. (*See also* Air pollutants and Ozone.)

Socioeconomic status
The social standing or class of an individual or group, typically measured by a combination of education, income, and occupation.

Stress
A condition, characterized by emotional or physical tension, which is a reaction to a situation that is threatening or otherwise causes feelings of anxiety.

Substance abuse
Taking illegal drugs or using too much alcohol, prescription medication, or other legal substances, or using them in the wrong way. Substance abuse

differs from addiction, a disease where one cannot stop using a substance even when its use is causing harm. (*See also* Addiction.)

Substance misuse
Use of a prescription drug for a purpose other than its intended purpose, or more generally, substance use that can cause harm to the user or their family or friends. (Some professionals believe that there is less stigma attached to this term than to the term "substance abuse.")

Thirdhand smoke
Tobacco smoke residue that settles on indoor surfaces and interacts with other indoor pollutants, creating a toxic mix of chemicals that may later become airborne.

Toxicant
A toxic substance created by human activity, such as an air pollutant or a pesticide. (*See also* Air pollutants, Air toxics, and Hazardous air pollutants.)

Toxicology
The study of how chemical, physical, and biological agents can adversely affect people, animals, and the environment.

Toxin
A toxic substance that is found in nature, such as snake venom or poisonous mushrooms.

Transpiration
The evaporation of water from plant, causing a cooling of the surrounding air.

Tsunami
A large ocean wave or series of waves that sometimes occurs following strong offshore earthquakes.

Ultraviolet (UV) radiation
Radiation from the sun that has been linked to skin cancer, premature aging, cataracts and other eye damage, and immune system suppression.

UV index
A forecast of the expected risk of overexposure to ultraviolet (UV) radiation from the sun, calculated by the National Weather Service and published by the U.S. Environmental Protection Agency (EPA).

Value chain
The process of adding value to raw materials through various processes at every production step to create a finished, marketable product.

Virus
A submicroscopic infective agent that grows and reproduces in living cells and is responsible for a wide range of infectious diseases.

Walk score
A number between 0 and 100 that measures the walkability of a city or any address, neighborhood, or ZIP code within the city, based on an analysis of (1) hundreds of walking routes to nearby amenities, and (2) pedestrian friendliness, taking into account population density and various road metrics. The website walkscore.com offers information about how to find the walk score of your community. (*See also* Bike score.)

Walkable neighborhood
When a person in reasonably good health can walk to nearby destinations without difficulty (e.g., visiting a grocery store, doctor's office, or park).

Withdrawal syndrome
A predictable group of signs and symptoms resulting from the abrupt decrease or removal of a psychoactive substance (e.g., a drug, alcohol, or nicotine).

Zoonotic disease
An infectious disease that is transmitted from animals to humans. Up to 60 percent of all infectious diseases in humans are zoonotic in origin. (*See also* Infectious disease.)

Directory of Resources

100 Resilient Cities

New York, NY

https://www.100resilientcities.org

100 Resilient Cities is a nonprofit organization supported by the Rockefeller Foundation that is dedicated to helping cities around the world become more resilient to the physical, social, and economic challenges that are a growing part of the twenty-first century. The organization supports the adoption of a view of resilience that helps cities respond to adverse events and deliver basic functions to all populations, in both good times and bad. Through this work, 100 Resilient Cities hopes to help individual cities become more resilient while facilitating the building of a global practice of resilience among governments, nongovernmental organizations, the private sector, and individual citizens.

Air and Waste Management Association (AWMA)

Pittsburgh, PA

https://www.awma.org

The Air and Waste Management Association (AWMA) is a professional organization dedicated to enhancing knowledge and expertise in the areas of air quality and waste management by providing a neutral forum for exchanging information. The AWMA provides professional development opportunities to its members, promotes global environmental responsibility, and helps organizations make critical decisions that benefit society. Many AWMA members are concerned with air and waste issues in urban areas, and its annual conference routinely includes urban topics, such as community health effects studies and air-quality monitoring.

American Cancer Society (ACS)

Atlanta, GA
https://www.cancer.org
The American Cancer Society is a nationwide, community-based, voluntary health organization dedicated to eliminating all forms of cancer. The society funds and conducts a wide range of research and provides advice on lifestyle, treatment, and recovery. Its website includes a summary of the latest recommendations from expert agencies on cell-phone use (https://www.cancer.org/cancer/cancer-causes/radiation-exposure/cellular-phones .html) and a review of cancer clusters sometimes found in urban areas (https://www.cancer.org/cancer/cancer-causes/general-info/cancer-clusters .html).

American Public Health Association (APHA)

Washington, DC
https://apha.org
The American Public Health Association (APHA) is a professional association with over 25,000 members representing virtually every field of public health and medicine. The programs supported by the APHA and its membership include healthy community design, community health planning and policy development, community-based public health, and smart growth (building healthy cities and neighborhoods that are economically prosperous, socially equitable, and environmentally sustainable).

Carter Center

Atlanta, GA
https://www.cartercenter.org
The Carter Center was founded by President Jimmy Carter and Rosalynn Carter as a nongovernmental organization to help advance peace and worldwide health by resolving global conflicts, advancing democracy and human rights, promoting economic opportunity, preventing diseases, improving mental health, and teaching farmers how to increase crop production. The

center has been particularly effective in reducing the incidence of infectious diseases in developing nations by improving disease surveillance and healthcare delivery systems. For communities burdened by several diseases, the center has pioneered public health approaches for treating multiple diseases at once.

Centers for Disease Control and Prevention (CDC)

Atlanta, GA
https://www.cdc.gov
The mission of the Centers for Disease Control and Prevention (CDC) is to protect Americans from health, safety, and security threats originating both in the United States and overseas. The CDC conducts research, provides health information to health agencies and the public, issues health alerts, and coordinates response activities with state and local agencies. The agency's National Center for Chronic Disease Prevention and Health Promotion (https://www.cdc.gov/chronicdisease/index.htm) funds programs that help communities promote healthy behaviors and reduce the major risk factors for chronic disease, such as tobacco use, lack of physical activity, and unhealthy eating. The CDC offers advice about the seasonal flu vaccination to protect against the flu (https://www.cdc.gov/flu/about/qa/flushot.htm). It also addresses health concerns regarding cell-phone use (https://www.cdc.gov/nceh/radiation/cell_phones._faq.html).

Environmental Protection Agency (EPA)

Washington, DC
https://www.epa.gov
The U.S. Environmental Protection Agency (EPA) is the nation's leading environmental agency for protecting human health and the environment. The EPA's priorities include developing and enforcing regulations, issuing research grants, studying environmental issues, sponsoring partnerships, teaching people about the environment, and protecting the rights of low-income and minority populations to a clean environment. A number of EPA initiatives concern the urban environment, including programs addressing healthy communities, community revitalization assistance, smart growth, urban waters, stormwater impacts, Superfund and brownfield sites, the urban heat island effect, environmental justice, and climate resilience.

The EPA ambient air-quality programs address smog and other air pollutants in urban areas, and the AirNow Air Quality Index (AQI; https://airnow.gov) reports air quality, including forecasts, for over 500 cities across the nation.

Food and Drug Administration (FDA)

Silver Spring, MD
https://www.fda.gov
The Food and Drug Administration (FDA) has a variety of responsibilities for protecting the safety of food and drugs in the United States. Additionally, the FDA ensures that vaccines and medical devices are safe and effective, protects the public from electronic product radiation, ensures that cosmetics and dietary supplements are safe and properly labeled, regulates tobacco products, and speeds up the pace of product innovation. The FDA estimates that there are almost 50 million foodborne illnesses annually in the United States, many in urban areas.

Health.gov

Washington, DC
https://health.gov
This website provides useful information on food and nutrition, physical activity, health literacy, and healthcare quality, including the U.S. government's latest dietary guidelines for healthy-eating patterns. The website is maintained by the U.S. Department of Health and Human Services, Office of Disease Prevention and Health Promotion.

Indian Health Service (IHS)

Rockville, MD
https://www.ihs.gov
The Indian Health Service, an agency within the U.S. Department of Health and Human Services, is the principal federal healthcare provider and health advocate for Native American and Alaska Native peoples. Its goal is to raise their health status to the highest possible level by ensuring that comprehensive and culturally acceptable personal and public health services are available to all communities.

Institute for Urban Health (IUH)

New York, NY
https://nyam.org/institute-urban-health
Located within the New York Academy of Medicine (https://nyam.org), the Institute for Urban Health is focused on finding multidimensional solutions for making cities healthier by integrating interdisciplinary research and evaluation, policy advocacy, and practice. Current work areas include healthy aging, disease prevention, and eliminating health disparities. The institute houses the Center for Health Policy and Programs, the Center for Cognitive Studies in Medicine and Public Health, the Center for Health Innovation, and the Center for Evaluation and Applied Research.

Intergovernmental Panel on Climate Change (IPCC)

Geneva, Switzerland
http://www.ipcc.ch
The Intergovernmental Panel on Climate Change (IPCC) is the world's leading international body for assessing the science related to climate change and providing the latest information to governments and policymakers. The IPCC conducts regular assessments of climate change science, impacts and future risks, and options for adaption and mitigation. Many of the IPCC's assessments are directed toward urbanization, including urban vulnerability, resilience, and adaption. A recent report discusses the rapid, far-reaching, and unprecedented changes in all aspects of society needed to limit climate change (http://www.ipcc.ch/report/sr15).

Journal of Urban Health

New York, NY
https://link.springer.com/journal/11524
The *Journal of Urban Health* (published by Springer US) offers research papers generally addressing the health and well-being of people in cities. According to the journal, it provides "a platform for interdisciplinary exploration of the evidence base for the broader determinants of health and health inequities needed to strengthen policies, programs, and governance for urban health." The journal is published six times annually.

Medical News Today

Brighton, East Sussex, UK
https://www.medicalnewstoday.com
Medical News Today, owned and operated by Healthline Media UK Ltd., is a leading publication concerned with developments in the medical field. One of its recent articles, "What Is Medicine? A History of Medicine" (https://www.medicalnewstoday.com/info/medicine), presents a good summary of the history of medicine, beginning with ancient Egypt.

National Academies of Sciences, Engineering, and Medicine (NASEM)

Washington, DC
http://www.nationalacademies.org
The National Academies of Sciences, Engineering, and Medicine is a private, nonprofit organization consisting of institutions that provide expert advice on some of the world's most challenging issues and that shape sound policies, inform public opinion, and advance the pursuit of science, engineering, and medicine. Its recent *Consensus Study Report: Public Health Consequences of E-cigarettes* (https://www.nap.edu/resource/24952/012318 ecigaretteHighlights.pdf) provides valuable information on e-cigarettes and vaping.

National Center for Complementary and Integrative Health (NCCIH)

Bethesda, MD
https://nccih.nih.gov
The National Center for Complementary and Integrative Health conducts research on diverse medical and healthcare systems, practices, and products that are not generally considered part of conventional medicine. Included in their purview are ancient practices, like Ayurvedic medicine, that continue to be practiced today in some parts of the world.

National Center for Environmental Health (NCEH)

Atlanta, GA
https://www.cdc.gov/nceh
The mission of the National Center for Environmental Health (NCEH) is to promote a healthy environment, prevent premature death, and help

people avoid illness and disability caused by environmental factors other than infectious disease agents and occupational exposures. The NCEH focuses particularly on vulnerable populations, such as children, older adults, and people with disabilities. Some programs cover topics of interest to urban dwellers, including asthma, childhood lead poisoning prevention, climate and health, food safety, natural disasters, and radiation emergencies.

National Institutes of Health (NIH)

Bethesda, MD

https://www.nih.gov

The National Institutes of Health (NIH) is the nation's leading medical research agency, with many of its programs at the forefront of global health protection. The NIH is made up of 27 separate institutes and centers, each having a specific research agenda concerning diseases, health challenges, and body systems. The National Institute on Alcohol Abuse and Alcoholism (https://www.niaaa.nih.gov), National Institute of Allergy and Infectious Diseases (https://www.niaid.nih.gov), National Institute on Drug Abuse (https://www.drugabuse.gov), National Institute of Environmental Health Sciences (niehs.nih.gov), National Institute on Minority Health and Health Disparities (https://www.nimhd.nih.gov), and several other NIH institutes conduct research on issues highly relevant to the urban environment.

National Oceanic and Atmospheric Administration (NOAA)

Washington, DC

http://www.noaa.gov

The mission of the National Oceanic and Atmospheric Administration (NOAA) is to conduct research, collect data, and disseminate information on the nation's climate, weather, oceans, and coasts. NOAA studies the structure and behavior of the oceans and atmosphere, conserves and manages coastal and marine ecosystems and resources, and responds to environmental emergencies. NOAA scientists study the effects of climate change (https://www.climate.gov), including the urban heat island effect, and NOAA weather forecasters, working under the National Weather Service, provide lifesaving information when natural disasters threaten urban areas, such as heat waves, floods, severe storms, and hurricanes.

Occupational Safety and Health Administration (OSHA)

Washington, DC
https://www.osha.gov
The mission of the Occupational Safety and Health Administration (OSHA) is to ensure that working Americans experience safe and healthful working conditions by implementing the requirements of the Occupational Safety and Health Act. OSHA sets and enforces standards, delivers training to employers and workers, and provides technical assistance. Because most new jobs in the United States are created in urban areas, many OSHA programs benefit the urban worker.

Organisation for Economic Cooperation and Development (OECD)

Paris, France
http://www.oecd.org
The Organisation for Economic Cooperation and Development (OECD) provides a forum for governments to cooperate in solving common problems, including the need for strong public health systems. The OECD's health program (http://www.oecd.org/els/health-systems/public-health.htm) addresses major risk factors of concern to urban dwellers, such as obesity, diet, physical activity, alcohol consumption, tobacco use, and environmental exposure. Additionally, it provides information on the spread of these risk factors in populations, including past and future trends, inequalities based on socioeconomic status, and the determinants underpinning risk factors. The OECD also publishes a health indicators report that provides information on the health status of populations and health-system performance in OECD member-states (http://www.oecd.org/health/health-systems).

United Nations (UN)

New York, NY
http://www.un.org
The United Nations takes action on the issues confronting humanity in the twenty-first century, such as peace and security, climate change, sustainable development, human rights, disarmament, terrorism, humanitarian and health emergencies, gender equality, governance, and food production. Its New Urban Agenda (http://habitat3.org/the-new-urban-agenda) presents a shared vision for the world community on creating a more sustainable future

where "all people have equal rights and access to the benefits and opportunities that cities can offer, and in which the international community reconsiders the urban systems and physical form of our urban spaces to achieve this." The United Nations also provides useful demographic and social statistics for urban areas (https://unstats.un.org/unsd/demographic-social).

Water Environment Federation (WEF)

Alexandria, VA
http://www.wef.org
The Water Environment Federation (WEF) is a professional organization representing over 33,000 individual members and 75 affiliated organizations around the world. The WEF's goals are to protect public health and the environment by enriching the experience of water pollution professionals, increasing public awareness about the importance of water, and providing a platform for innovation. Many members are concerned with water quality and sanitation issues in urban areas, including the need for improved water-quality education and training in developing nations.

World Health Organization (WHO)

Geneva, Switzerland
http://www.who.int
The World Health Organization (WHO) provides global leadership on matters critical to human health by shaping the global research agenda, setting norms and standards, articulating ethical and evidence-based policies, providing technical support, and monitoring health trends. The WHO sponsors initiatives and provides information on urban health (http://www .who.int/topics/urban_health), urban population growth (http://www.who .int/gho/urban_health/situation_trends/urban_population_growth), global age-friendly cities (http://www.who.int/ageing/projects/age_friendly_cities), and water and sanitation in healthcare facilities (http://www.who.int/water _sanitation_health/publications/wash-health-care-facilities/en). WHO's Center for Health Development (http://www.who.int/kobe_centre/about) includes programs on measuring urban health, interventions on urban health, urban health emergencies, and aging. Its International Agency for Research on Cancer addresses the facts about cell-phone use and health (http://www.who.int/news-room/fact-sheets/detail/electromagnetic-fields -and-public-health-mobile-phones).

Index

Note: Page numbers followed by *t* indicate tables and *f* indicate figures.

About the Author

Richard V. Crume is a consultant, educator, and journalist with more than 40 years of professional experience managing environmental health programs, conducting research in the environmental sciences, and teaching university classes on air pollution and climate change. He serves on the American Public Health Association's Governing Council and wrote their national policy statement on air quality. Additionally, Crume belongs to the National Association of Science Writers, the Society of Environmental Journalists, and the Institute of Professional Environmental Practice (Qualified Environmental Professional Emeritus). In recognition of his contributions to the environmental health field, Crume was awarded the U.S. Environmental Protection Agency's Gold Medal for Excellence and the agency's Suzanne E. Olive Award for Exemplary Leadership. He is the editor of Greenwood's *Environmental Health in the 21st Century: From Air Pollution to Zoonotic Diseases.*